THE UNTAPPED SELF

GERAD KITE
& JAMES EDEN

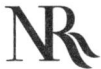

Published in 2025 by New River Books
Unit 105, Leroy House, 436 Essex Road, London N1 3QP
www.newriverbooks.co.uk

10 9 8 7 6 5 4 3 2 1

Copyright © Gerad Kite and James Eden 2025

Gerad Kite and James Eden have asserted their rights under the Copyright, Designs and Patents Act 1988 to be identified as the authors of this work. All rights reserved. No part of this publication may be reproduced, stored in a retrieval system or transmitted in any form, or by any means (electronic, mechanical, or otherwise) without the prior written permission of both the copyright owners and the publisher.

A CIP catalogue record for this book is available from the British Library.

ISBN: 978-1-915780-41-6

Printed and Bound in the UK using 100% Renewable Electricity at CPI Group (UK) Ltd, Croydon, CR0 4YY.

Cover design: Jo Walker
Interior cover design: Peagreen

This FSC® label means that materials used for the product have been responsibly sourced.

CONTENTS

Introduction: Rushing into the Middle	4
1. Broken Bowl	27
2. Illuminated Sea	56
3. Loathsome Jaw	86
4. Welcome Fragrance	111
5. Listening Palace	135
6. Earth Motivator	161
7. Fly and Scatter	189
8. Palace of Weariness	213
9. Walk Between	243
10. Very Great Abyss	275
Epilogue	300
Glossary	302

INTRODUCTION

RUSHING INTO THE MIDDLE

*

Not long after my twenty-fifth birthday, my life began to unravel. From the outside, everything looked great. I was newly married, I had become a partner in a thriving business and I was beginning to carve out a new life in San Francisco. Behind the shiny façade, however, all was not well. My marriage was a sham, I was chronically depressed and my substance abuse was bordering on addiction. In the space of a few short months, the life that I had begun to build for myself in the land of opportunity came tumbling down.

I had arrived in the United States a year earlier, the result of a decision that I had made when I was drunk. I had been running a travel business in London with a man who I was madly in love with. Unfortunately, despite the sexual tension that I felt, our relationship remained platonic. The sadness and frustration were overwhelming, but rather than confront the situation, I dealt with it in the only way I knew how to – passive aggression and workaholism by day, alcohol abuse by night. Our partnership became fractured and untenable until one day, without so much as a word, he picked up his things and left. Nine months later, I was still reeling from his departure but I didn't feel that I could tell anyone how I was feeling. One evening, as I sat at my desk polishing off a bottle of wine, my eyes were drawn to a business card propped up against my pen holder. It had been left by an American woman who had visited me earlier that year after reading about our business in the *New York Times*. "You should come to California," she had told me. "I think you and I would work well together." Emboldened by the alcohol, I picked up the phone and dialled her number. A month later, having shut down the business that I had worked so hard to create, I was on a plane to America.

San Francisco was exhilarating and terrifying in equal measure. The city was in the throes of the dot com boom but the remnants of its Bohemian past were everywhere to be seen. Hair was long, skirts were short, and the sweet smell of marijuana lingered outside the cafés and bookshops that were holding out as long as they could against the unstoppable wave of change. Yet my abiding memory is neither the laid-back hippies nor the fast-living entrepreneurs. It is the sight of emaciated young men walking the streets of the Castro district with hollow eyes and walking sticks, hapless victims of a merciless epidemic for which there was no cure. In the months that followed, I discovered that lacing your orange juice with MDMA was the norm, that what you did and where you came from didn't matter, and that everyone knew somebody who had died of AIDS. I was in a city full of renegades and runaways, a hedonistic paradise where anything was possible, if only you could stay alive long enough to make it happen. By day I made money, lots of it. By night I hung out with my friends as we tried in vain to make sense of ourselves and our lives through the fog of drink and drugs.

I had entered the United States on a short-term tourist visa, and a few months into my stay, I realised that, unless I was granted an extension, I would have to leave the country or risk being deported. The thought of returning to England was unbearable and I fell into a depression. Then one evening, my neighbour appeared at my door clutching a potato and asked if she could use my oven. In the hour it took for the potato to bake, Beth and I had drunk a bottle of tequila, put the world to rights and had sex. At that time, sexual orientation was largely irrelevant and even though I didn't consciously identify as bisexual, Beth and I quickly became a couple. We got on like a house on fire, and a few months later, spurred on by my visa situation, we stood on the steps of City Hall as man and wife. My future in California seemed to have been sealed.

Our decadent existence continued unabated and it was not long before Beth announced that she was pregnant. I was over the moon at first, but then reality hit. At the tender age of twenty, Beth would soon be a mother. What had started as a drug-fuelled marriage of convenience was destined to become a lifelong commitment. I was utterly conflicted. I loved Beth and the more conventional part of me wanted nothing more than to become a father, but the thought of signing up for a monogamous, heterosexual marriage was more than I could bear. So my confused, fearful, twenty-five-year-old self contrived to find a way out. After much discussion and heartache, we agreed to terminate the pregnancy, but to my eternal shame, I was not honest. Gripped by the fear of being trapped in a situation which, instinctively, felt contrary to my nature, I steered the decision in the direction that I wanted, using our age and our substance abuse as an excuse. There was some truth in it, but my driving motivation above all was to come to terms with my sexuality and accept that having a conventional family life was not on the cards. Shortly after the termination, I began to withdraw my affection, and it wasn't long before I told Beth that I wanted to end the marriage. To this day, I bitterly regret the way I handled the situation, and the gnawing pain of having relinquished the chance to be a father endures.

My dishonesty gave me back my freedom, but the trade was hard. I was overwhelmed by guilt and loneliness, and my mental and physical health began to deteriorate. My gums bled profusely and each night felt like the dark night of the soul as I thrashed around, drenched in sweat, desperately trying to find some inner peace. Until this point in my life, I had always found a way to suppress my more uncomfortable emotions. In fact, it was nothing more than a coping mechanism, born of a belief formed during my childhood that weakness was not to be tolerated. I prided myself on being the strong one, the person that everyone turned to in times of trouble. Now, all of a sudden, the strategy didn't work any more. I kept my suffering private for as long as I could, but eventually my pride gave way to humility. I was in freefall and I knew that if something didn't change my life would spiral out of control, so I reached out to one of my closest friends for help.

"You should go and see an acupuncturist," she told me. "I know just the person."

"Are you serious?" I replied. "How on earth can an acupuncturist help me?"

"Go see him and you'll find out."

There was a time in my life when the idea of visiting an acupuncturist would have been met with a snort of derision, but I was desperate. The following week, I found myself sitting opposite a middle-aged man with soft brown eyes and an air of wisdom. His name was Emmett and he had been practising Five-Element Acupuncture since his early thirties. He began by asking me about myself, but I found it almost impossible to answer his questions. It felt as though he were speaking a foreign language. He persisted, and before long I began to express myself in a way that had been completely alien to me until that moment. When we finished talking, he led me to the treatment table and started to work his magic. To begin with, he took my hand and began to apply a light pressure to my wrists with his fingertips. He was, as I would come to discover, taking the Chinese pulses. Then he got to work with the needles. Lying there that day, feeling the gentle touch of another human being as the glowing aftermath of the acupuncture treatment swept through my body, I felt hopeful and uplifted.

That night I slept soundly and awoke feeling calm. As

I sat in the window smoking my first cigarette of the day, I noticed a woman looking up at me from the back of a bus in the street below. As our eyes met, she smiled at me as if to say, "Everything's OK", and somehow in that moment I knew that it was. In the weeks that followed, I saw Emmett regularly, and the effects of the treatments were dramatic. Little by little, the scales fell from my eyes. I felt as though I were watching a movie in which I was the protagonist, struggling to deal with conflicting emotions that were wrestling for control. At the time, it didn't occur to me that this objective point of perception could be the outcome of the acupuncture treatment. Nevertheless, my entire outlook on life began to change and, quite unexpectedly, I felt an overwhelming compulsion to return to the UK. My time in San Francisco had been a whirlwind of excitement, but it had also taken its toll. It was time to leave, and once again, just as I had done the year before, I packed my bags and boarded a plane.

A few days after arriving home, I went to see an old family friend, a vivacious Irish lady called Anne who worked as a psychotherapist. "Oh, my Lord, aren't you just the luckiest man in the world!" she exclaimed when I told her about my experience. "You've woken up!" I was still oscillating between states of sadness and joy, but Anne's reaction was so disarmingly positive that for a few precious moments, any residual angst fell away.

"So what do I do now?"

"What do you do? The only thing that's worth doing in this life. You learn about yourself. And then you learn about others."

"But how?" I asked. Anne pulled a stack of papers from her desk and pressed them into my hands.

"These are from the Pellin Institute. I studied psychotherapy there with a man called Peter Fleming. Ask him if he will teach you. I think you're ready."

Within a month of arriving back in the UK, I had enrolled at the Pellin Institute and was immersing myself in the strange new world of Gestalt psychology and Contribution Training. I was proud of myself for having taken the leap, but I was ill-prepared. I was one of ten students, and at the beginning of each session, we would take it in turns to speak. Interruptions were forbidden. I was bored and irritated and, having been effectively gagged, all I could do was listen to the contents of my mind, a chaos of groundless judgements and preconceptions. I thought about quitting but Anne's words kept ringing in my ears and eventually I surrendered to the process. Little by little, I began to take responsibility for the thoughts in my head and the way that they coloured my experience. It was my first real taste of self-awareness.

Before I left San Francisco, Emmett had given me one of his business cards, on the back of which he had written the name and number of an acupuncturist in London, and two words: SEDATE WOOD. And so, a month or so after arriving back in London, I jumped in my little green car and made my way to Notting Hill. Madelaine was glamorous and motherly, and she made delicious soup. After a few sessions, I asked her what Emmett had meant by SEDATE WOOD.

"Sedate Wood? Well, Emmett's diagnosis was that your

Wood element is out of balance. The organs that relate to Wood are the liver and the gallbladder, and it seems that yours are very agitated, so I need to calm them down." She popped four needles in both of my feet and then took my pulses. "You see, we're all composed of the same five elements that we see in the natural world. Wood, Fire, Earth, Metal and Water. We think we're separate beings but we're not. We're a part of Nature, just like everything else. And if you look carefully, you can see that we follow the same laws and rhythms." I gave her a quizzical look and she beamed at me. "The ancient Chinese knew that the liver is the only organ in the body that can regenerate itself, just like the trees and plants in the spring. The Western world only worked that out at the beginning of the twentieth century. Isn't that amazing?"

I was immediately captivated by the magic of this system of medicine. It had a simple but profound logic, and a seductive ring of truth that I found irresistible. I visited Madelaine regularly, and each time I became a little more intrigued by what she was doing. Sensing my interest, she told me about two renowned sinologists, Claude Larre and Elisabeth Rochat de la Vallée, who gave weekly lectures on the ancient Chinese medical texts. I was anxious to learn more about this mysterious art, so each week I made my way to Covent Garden and, little by little, the seed that had been planted by my first acupuncture treatment began to take root.

One gloomy afternoon in early autumn, I visited Madelaine and told her that, although I found the psychotherapy training interesting, I couldn't see myself making it my profession. "Something's missing," I told her.

"So why don't you study acupuncture?" she replied. "You clearly love it." I had often gazed at her graduation certificate on the wall and marvelled that she was already ten years into her practice.

"You really think I could do this?"

"Of course! What are you waiting for?"

I walked out of Madelaine's clinic that day with a spring in my step. Just like that, my life had taken another unexpected turn.

* * *

On a bright, sunny day in September 1989, I walked into the College of Traditional Acupuncture in Royal Leamington Spa for my first day as a student of acupuncture. I had expected my fellow students to be Oxbridge intellectuals in shirts and skirts, but instead I found myself surrounded by a group of middle-aged men and women who looked as if they belonged in the Peace Corps. On the first morning, we learned about the history of Chinese medicine and I quickly realised that this ancient tradition was still every bit as relevant as it was when it had first emerged three thousand years earlier. I learned that Taoism and Five-Element Acupuncture belong to a spiritual tradition and system of medicine whose concern is to maintain the balance of body, mind and spirit. It is this fundamental equilibrium that enables us to enjoy a peaceful and harmonious life. The part that really caught my attention, though, was how this philosophy explains our unique responses to the world and to each other. Until this point, I had rarely questioned the origin of my thoughts, emotions and actions. I had had brief glimpses of self-awareness in the psychotherapy training in London, but most of the time I led a fairly compulsive and blinkered existence. All of a sudden, I was being presented with a philosophy that explained myself, those around me and our reactions to one another with a seemingly irrefutable logic. The next lecture laid out the theory that underpins the practice of acupuncture.

"The entire universe is made up of one vital life force called 'qi', which manifests as five distinct elements," we were told. The lecturer picked up a blue crayon, drew a large circle on the bottom left corner of the blackboard and coloured it in. She turned to see our reaction. Blank faces stared back at her. "The Water element!" she declared. She drew four more circles. Green for Wood, red for Fire, yellow for Earth and white for Metal. A circle of circles. Finally she added clockwise arrows to connect the five elements and a pentagonal star in the centre. "Each of us is made up of the five elements. When all five are correctly interconnected and balanced, order is maintained. When there is an imbalance, our entire system is thrown into disarray and distress signals appear in the form of symptoms." The penny dropped. It was so simple that a child of five could have understood it.

By the end of the lecture, I had a basic understanding of each of the five elements. The Wood element, I had learned, governs our capacity to be born and reborn. Its associated season is spring, the time when new life rises from the depths of winter, giving us a sense of hope and excitement for the future. Wood gives us the capacity to see our potential and the roadmap to realise it. The Fire element, which is associated with the height of summer, gives us the capacity to love and be loved. It governs the circulatory system, bringing warmth to every part of our being, nurturing communication and intimacy, and enabling us to be at ease with our ever-changing internal and external environment. The Earth element is the flesh on our bones. It is associated with late summer, the time when the fruits of the earth are harvested and stored away to give us a sense of security and contentment. The Earth element provides us with a stable foundation from which to navigate our lives, and a sense of belonging that comes from the capacity to maintain a reciprocal relationship with the world around us. The Metal element, which is associated with autumn, is the destructive part of the cycle, the counterbalance to the creative force of the Wood element that is seen in spring. It gives us the capacity to know what is of most value for our body, mind and spirit. Anything that is not needed is discarded. Finally, there is the mighty Water element, the origin of all life, which is associated with the season of winter. This is the element that gives us power and reassurance; the innate sense that we have all that we need to survive. The Water element governs the flow of our physical form, our emotional states and our spiritual evolution; it operates all levels of our being, giving us the capacity to move with ease between stillness and movement.

RUSHING INTO THE MIDDLE

* * *

Two months into my acupuncture training, there was a buzz of excitement as I entered the school. "JR's teaching this week!" one of my fellow students shouted as she ran down the corridor. JR Worsley was a legend in the acupuncture world. After studying in Asia with two Chinese masters in the late fifties, he had brought Five-Element Acupuncture to the West and in 1979, after a period teaching in the United States, opened the College of Traditional Acupuncture in Leamington Spa. People talked about this man with such excitement and respect that the thought of him teaching us in person was the highlight of the year. JR's charismatic presence was matched by his sartorial elegance. Whenever I saw him, he was immaculately turned out in a three-piece suit and white shirt, occasionally finished off with a bow tie, which added to his professorial aura. From time to time, he would inject a bit of humour into the proceedings but the seriousness of what he was teaching was never in question. In fact, I always felt that the way he dressed was a reflection of his reverence for the ancient knowledge and wisdom that he was passing on to another generation of would-be practitioners. His lecture that day was on the 'Causative Factor', the name given to the element that is the original cause of all imbalance in the patient's body, mind *and* spirit. The Causative Factor is the cornerstone of this system of medicine and the foundation on which our entire approach to treatment is built.

"Pay careful attention," he warned us. "A person's

symptoms, be they mental, physical or spiritual, are of no help to us whatsoever. They are nothing but distress signals coming from one or more of the five elements. Our job is to find the root of the problem, and this is what we call the Causative Factor." He wrote the letters 'CF' on the blackboard, removed his glasses with a theatrical flourish and turned to face us. "And it's damned hard to find." He paused for a moment to let his words sink in and then continued. "Every day you will get better and better at finding the Causative Factor but I'll warn you now, you are going to have to work at this for the rest of your life."

The following afternoon, I walked into the classroom to find a teacher wearing baggy trousers, sandals and a cloth cap. The contrast with JR was striking.

"Yesterday, JR told you about the Causative Factor, or the CF as we like to call it. Today I am going to teach you how to diagnose it. Every single person on the face of this planet has a CF. It is the unique cause of every imbalance in their body, mind and spirit and it does not change throughout their lifetime. The CF is the element in each person that is in trouble, creating problems not only for itself but for the other four elements as well. By diagnosing and treating the CF, we help Nature restore balance and harmony." She turned to face the blackboard and wrote four words in big white letters: COLOUR, SOUND, ODOUR, EMOTION. "Let me make this easy for you. Nature is the healer, and you are its instrument. The moment the causal element goes out of balance, Nature sends out one unified distress signal, which is received in four different ways by the practitioner – an unusual *colour* in the face, a jarring *sound* in the voice, a distinctive *odour* and an inappropriate *emotion*. All you have to do is pay attention to what Nature is telling you. Nature will lead you to the cause."

The gauntlet had been laid down but, as ready as I was for a challenge, I was struggling to quieten both the voice of scepticism and the fear of failure that were ringing in my ears. Diagnose someone's illness by their odour? Really? For as long as I could remember, I had lived my life from a rigidly subjective standpoint, judging, analysing and labelling everything according to firmly entrenched patterns and beliefs. Now, I was being asked to set aside my rational mind and tap into an altogether different part of myself. I went home that day wondering if I had it in me to complete the training, but when morning came, I awoke with a renewed sense of optimism and determination to succeed.

Each week, I set myself the task of exploring one of the four pillars of diagnosis. Our teachers had told us that the best way to become attuned to the senses was to be in nature, so on the morning of the first week, I headed out to the park and lay beneath a large ash tree. To begin with, all I could see was a uniform green colour, but as the week progressed, I began to notice the subtle differences in the leaves. The more I relaxed, the more I could see. Week number two was sound, and eavesdropping became my new hobby. Wherever I went, I closed my eyes and listened to whatever was unfolding. At first, it was almost impossible not to get caught up in what people were saying, but eventually I learned to focus my full attention on the sound in their voices. Little by little, patterns emerged, distinct tones and rhythms that repeated over and over again. Week three was odour. To their consternation, I began greeting friends and family with a prolonged hug, surreptitiously sniffing them as I did so. My inner sceptic convinced me that all I would be able to smell was perfume or sweat, but soon enough I began to notice that everyone has their own unique odour. My fourth and final task was to feel other people's emotions and, just as I had imagined, it was the toughest challenge of them all. I knew how *I* felt when I was with someone, but how on earth could I know what *they* were feeling? Little did I know that the question contained the answer. For the first few days, I struggled. Then, slowly but surely, I learned something extraordinary. The way we are truly able to know how another person is feeling is not by interpreting their outward appearance, which can be misleading, but by remaining neutral and paying attention to the way that being in their presence makes *us* feel.

The tasks I had set for myself during those four weeks dramatically changed my attitude towards what I was learning. Week after week, my senses had begun to come alive and I finally understood what our teachers had been telling us: in this system of medicine, a diagnosis isn't the outcome of an objective evaluation. It is the result of sensory perception and experience, and that happens inside us. It would take time for my senses to become sufficiently attuned to make reliable diagnoses but, in the meantime, the way that I perceived the world had begun to change and my resistance had given way to curiosity.

In the years that followed, I learned about the powers, virtues, climates, flavours and emotions of each of the five elements. It was an encyclopaedia of knowledge that not only explained the cycles of Nature, but also the way in which we manifest in this world. It was, quite simply, a map of the human condition. No less extraordinary was the way in which the ancient Chinese had visualised the human body as an intricate network of energetic channels, known as 'meridians', through which 'qi', the life force in all things, is received, transformed and distributed. Most astonishing of all was the discovery that the meridians don't exist per se: they are the spaces in between everything. As unconventional as all of this was, it was starting to make perfect sense to me.

Another thing that I found particularly striking was the recognition that every organism requires its constituent parts to work together as one. If any individual part ceases to function as it should, the failure has an immediate effect on the entire system. The ancient Chinese observed this not only in the human body, but also in the natural world and the society in which they lived. It was this fundamental recognition that provided the foundation for this system of medicine. The organs and functions of the body, mind and spirit were likened to the officials of a kingdom, and were named as such. Each official had its own distinct role, but also worked for the success of the whole.

In the West, the organs of the body are thought of

purely in terms of their physiological function, whereas in ancient China they were believed to operate on all three levels of being – body, mind and spirit. For example, the Liver official is not only the physical organ; it also regulates the smooth flow of energy and, amongst many other things, it gives us the ability to formulate a vision for the future. Similarly, the Stomach official is responsible not only for the digestion of food, but also for providing stability and the capacity to think.

The more I learned about the officials, the more I fell in love with them. The Large Intestine, which is known as the "drainer of the dregs", is responsible for identifying and eliminating everything that we no longer need, be it the contents of our bowels, lingering resentments, or even attachment to the memory of those we have lost. Similarly, learning that the Lung was known as the "receiver of the heavenly qi" fundamentally changed the way I thought about breathing. Little by little, I began to learn that most of what I took for granted was an integral part of the sophisticated and beautiful expression of all life.

The jewel in the crown of my training was the so-called Spirit of the Points. In ancient China, almost all of the acupuncture points were given a name that describes unique human qualities. For example, our capacity to be decisive, to feel compassion, to find purpose in what we do, or carry out basic physiological functions. The names of the points are at times poetic, at times literal, but they all convey the possibility of awakening the extraordinary faculties that all too often lie dormant within us. One of my favourite teachers had a wonderful knack of describing the points in a simple, practical and humorous way, but he never failed to convey their spiritual significance. "Lubrication Food Gate is a point found on the Stomach meridian," he told us in one of his first lectures. "As it says on the tin, this point lubricates your digestive tract to ensure smooth digestion and evacuation." With a deadpan expression, he lifted his leg and made the sound of someone passing wind. "The richness of life is constantly moving through us. Everything we experience, without exception, is absorbed by us on one level or another. Listening to music, eating a meal, feeling the suffering of another. Every single experience nourishes us and enables us to appreciate the full experience of being human. Just imagine if this capacity within you stopped working. Nothing would move and nothing would be absorbed. You would no longer be nourished by your experience. Can you imagine how that would make you feel?"

* * *

Entering the world of Five-Element Acupuncture had given me a new lease of life and taken the edge off my sadness, yet the peace I yearned for still eluded me. I had the feeling that if only I could peel back the layers of confusion, there would eventually be an 'Aha!' moment when everything would suddenly make sense. I would find peace with my past and present and live happily ever after. That never happened. During my time of crisis, I had devoured every self-help book I could find, searching for ways to heal myself. Louise Hay and her philosophy of self-love was a favourite of mine. It posed a very simple question: "What is stopping you from loving yourself?" I liked myself, but love? That was a stretch. I was afraid that I was delusional. Had I done something terribly wrong that I couldn't remember? Did I unconsciously harbour a deep sense of self-loathing that would prevent me from healing myself? I tried all sorts of different therapies but the moment of revelation never came. Sure, I connected the dots of my history and there were even some revelations along the way, but did anything fundamentally change? No. In fact, a lot of what I had been told didn't ring true. For example, it was implied that having not witnessed a loving relationship between my parents, I would therefore struggle to form long-term relationships of my own. It was a convenient explanation, but if it were true how was it that my sister was happily married? What I did learn about myself was that the constant, nagging discomfort that I had felt for most of my life – a deep, painful, heartbroken kind of sadness – was not normal. When things were going well, I was happily distracted from it, but often it would be exacerbated by feelings of loneliness, rejection or betrayal. I thought this was how everyone felt, but in my final year of acupuncture training that assumption was finally put to rest when I had the opportunity to be diagnosed by JR himself.

Right from my very first acupuncture treatment with Emmett, I had been treated on the Wood element and I had convinced myself that this diagnosis defined me in some way. Depending on the circumstances, I would either use it as a badge of honour or a way to excuse my behaviour. In retrospect, it was laughable, but we all love labels, even if they are self-limiting. When JR changed my diagnosis to the Fire element, I was shocked. It felt like someone had just changed my name or given me a new star sign, but it turned out to be a transformational moment in my understanding of this system of medicine and, indeed, of myself. I realised that we are beyond definitions, that being part of Nature is to be a cog in the machinery of a constantly evolving universe and that labels – all labels – were nonsense. So what was the significance of this new diagnosis? Well, in truth it was simply that it helped my practitioner to know how best to help me. It was a signpost. Sure, it gave me an insight into the way in which I struggled, but it didn't explain *why* I struggled, and to think that it did was to lapse into a self-limiting mindset. Fire was not a definition; it simply pointed to the cause of imbalance in all five of the elements of which I am made. The acupuncture treatment that I received that day affected me in a way that nothing else, other than the fleeting joy of falling in love, had ever done before. I remember feeling the cold stone of sadness that had been my constant companion dissolve and a lightness begin to flow through me. After the session, I ran out of the school and jumped into my friend's car.

"Your face is bright red!" she said. "What's going on?"

"I have choice," I replied.

To this day, I am not entirely sure what I meant by that, but the word 'choice' emerged from a feeling of confidence and happiness that I had not experienced since childhood. It wasn't a conclusion reached through intellectual enquiry or experience. It was the outcome of an effortless return to a natural state of being, a knowing without cause or rationale. When I think of the most memorable events of my life, I was either head over heels in love or suffering from a feeling of rejection and betrayal. At no point had it occurred to me that my reactions were either inappropriate or extreme; nor did it occur to me that I could choose to behave any differently. In fact, it was the volatility of an unbalanced Fire element, my Achilles heel, if you like, that had produced these extremes. If I could find my way back to balance, the way in which I behaved and the choices I made would be of my own volition rather than the result of unconscious impulses. This realisation was shocking to me. No longer could I berate other people for their lack of enthusiasm or blame them for making me feel hurt and sad. The way I felt was entirely my own responsibility. This discovery set me on a totally new path. I realised that maintaining the midpoint, the steady and reliable inner warming of the Fire, was far more important than pursuing the fleeting pleasures to be found in the outside world. As JR used to say to us, "To love and be loved. That is the gift of Fire."

'Rushing into the Middle' is an acupuncture point on one of the Fire meridians located at the end of the middle finger, furthest away from the heart. It gives us the capacity to open our hearts to the world with love and engage fully with the gifts of life. It is a fundamentally human capacity, yet so many of us struggle to find it within.

RUSHING INTO THE MIDDLE

* * *

In the autumn of 1992, I graduated from the College of Traditional Acupuncture. Four years after my dark night of the soul, I had somehow managed to transform myself from a dispirited, hopeless young man into a qualified psychotherapist and Five-Element acupuncturist with a palpable sense of purpose. The story of my life before I found my path is by no means unique. On the contrary, it is a story as old as time. I set out to gain the world and in the process, I lost my connection with what really matters. Thankfully, I was given a second chance.

Throughout my thirty-five years of practice, I have been granted a rare and privileged window into the lives of my patients. To bring my learning to life, I teamed up with my trusted friend and co-author, James Eden, whose deep appreciation for Eastern philosophy, combined with his wonderful use of language, played a pivotal role in shaping the narrative of this book. Together, we set out to transform my experience into a collection of patient stories that capture the mystery and majesty of this ancient tradition in a way that would resonate for a contemporary audience.

But why stories? Throughout its long history, Five-Element Acupuncture has been passed down from master to apprentice and, as with all great oral traditions, storytelling lies at its heart. Stories have the ability to transcend boundaries, and I believe there is no better way to transmit this timeless wisdom than through the experiences of those who have felt its transformative power. All of the stories in this book are based on real patients who, like me, were searching for a way to heal themselves. However, in order to respect confidentiality, they have been heavily disguised. Each chapter features a composite character, carefully crafted from the experiences of numerous patients who share a similar diagnosis. Together, they illustrate the different ways in which many of us struggle, and the transformation that can take place within us when the natural order is restored. The treatments described are not representative of the entire clinical intervention that I would have made in each case. Rather, they are designed to give you a flavour of this ancient art.

As you read the stories that follow, I invite you to reflect on the profound healing potential that they reveal. We all face moments of disconnection and imbalance in our lives, yet the possibility of restoration and renewal is always there. I encourage you to embrace the wisdom of this ancient tradition and consider how it can support your own path to healing. For some people, the change can be dramatic; for others, less so, but the promise for all of us is a reconnection with our true nature. As we regain our state of balance, the untapped self begins to emerge, paving the way for an entirely new way of being.

1

BROKEN BOWL

*

My first encounter with Tor was a little odd, which is just the way I like it. In my world, everything is information. The stranger the interaction, the swifter the diagnosis. It was late August and, after a brief attempt at summer, London was once again conforming to its stereotype. It had been dry when I left home but as I emerged from the tube, it was chucking it down. I pulled my jacket over my head and headed west along Marylebone Road before turning into Wimpole Street. I stood for a moment on the steps of my clinic, watching the raindrops bounce off the pavement before gathering into miniature rapids that swept away the previous day's debris. I shook the rain from my jacket, took a deep breath to release my irritation and pushed open the door.

"Good morning, Gerad. Your first patient is here." The voice belonged to the receptionist, Eszter, a Hungarian woman in her early fifties whose brusque manner and fierce expression were curiously at odds with her chosen profession. I loved her, not least because the way in which she announced the arrival of a patient always told me something useful about the person I was shortly to encounter.

"She's been here for twenty minutes already," she continued, raising her eyes to the ceiling. "She asked if I had a watering can."

"A watering can?" I'm always excited to meet a new patient. Making a diagnosis is one of the things I love most about my work and it starts from the very first moment that I set eyes on someone. I turned towards the waiting room and stopped just short of the open doorway. To my left, a middle-aged man with half-moon spectacles was filling out a form while a nervous-looking girl sat quietly by his side. All of the other chairs were unoccupied, but on the far side of the room, the contents of a brightly coloured patchwork bag had been emptied over the sofa: an empty yoghurt pot, a half-eaten banana, a screwdriver and a dilapidated Filofax stuffed full of receipts. Someone had made a nest. I leaned forward and peered around the doorway. To my right was an open window, out of which the uncomfortably thin figure of a woman was leaning, one leg slightly raised to extend her reach and maintain her balance. I coughed into my hand but there was no reaction, so I stepped closer to the window to make sure that I was within earshot.

"Good morning, I believe you're here to see me." The woman ducked her head beneath the window and turned to face me. She was dressed in an orange jumpsuit and a long silk cardigan the colour of a parakeet. Her hair was swept back to reveal a pair of circular wooden earrings, and she had deep-set brown eyes that were bereft of sparkle, framed by temples that gave off a yellowish hue. In her right hand was an empty plastic cup that she held aloft.

"The flowers," she said, by way of an explanation. "They need water."

I glanced outside at the rain. "They do?"

"It's just a shower. You can never be too careful."

I smiled and held out my hand. "I'm Gerad."

Her face lit up. "Tell me, Gerad, why is it that people don't look after their window boxes? Everywhere you go, it's the same. Plants gasping for water. If I had my way, I'd set them all free." Her speech was like a lullaby, rhythmic and lilting, drawing me in with every word. She tossed the plastic cup in the bin and took my hand. "I'm Tor. It's Victoria, actually, but who wants to be named after a train station?" I tried to release my hand but it was stuck fast. "I really need your help, Gerad," she said, looking into my eyes with a pleading expression.

"Of course," I said, peeling my hand away. "That's what I'm here for."

"You see, I'm fifteen weeks pregnant and… Well, I'm desperately worried that I won't be allowed to keep it." For a split second, I froze. In front of me stood a woman who was so emaciated that her clothes hung off her, yet she had just told me that she was almost four months pregnant. Not only that, but she seemed to be suggesting that the pregnancy was in jeopardy. It was not the kind of disclosure I would expect someone to make in such a public place.

"Come with me and you can tell me everything in private. You're a little early but if you don't mind waiting…" Tor slowly returned the contents of her nest to the bag and lifted it over her shoulder, exhaling audibly with the effort. I gestured for her to follow me and, as we walked down the narrow staircase, I kept looking behind me in case she stumbled. Barely a minute had passed but a number of significant things had already caught my attention. The garish clothes, the sound of her voice, the firm handshake, the desperation in her eyes. All of it spoke volumes. This was a woman who wanted my full attention and, like it or not, I was going to give it to her. "Can I get you a glass of water?"

"What I'd really like is a hot lemon and honey. Could you do that for me?" It was a question but I sensed that it was non-negotiable. I walked to the adjoining kitchen feeling strangely agitated and rummaged through the cupboards looking for some honey. We hadn't even started the consultation but already everything felt very odd. I wondered if her friends and family felt like this around her or whether my reaction to her was a result of my own personal triggers. Not allowing my feelings to encroach on my objective observations of someone I've just met can be quite a challenge, but it is essential if I am to make an accurate diagnosis. In the Five-Element tradition, we call this being an 'instrument of Nature' and it is one of the things that makes my work so compelling and liberating. No matter what's going on in my own life, the moment I step into the role of the practitioner, my point of perception shifts and my attention goes to what I experience through my senses. I enter a state in which the 'I' with judgements, preferences and personal reactions takes a back seat. The 'I' that remains observes what is happening from a place of peace and neutrality. Whatever disturbs this peace is what catches my attention and leads me to the source of my patients' problems. When I started out in my early thirties, I found it almost impossible to do, but over time it has become second nature. During the first few minutes with a new patient, preconceptions and judgements abound, but as soon as the session begins, the personal mind is banished and the senses awaken.

I returned to the room, mug in hand, to find that she had removed her sandals and was now sitting cross-legged on the chair. I handed her the hot drink, took my seat and scribbled the date on a blank sheet of paper.

"Welcome, Tor."

"Thank you." She raised the mug to her lips and took a sip. "Hmm. It's a little sweet." Our relationship had begun.

* * *

Tor was forty-four and full of contradictions. Her speech was that of a sophisticated woman, yet her demeanour was reminiscent of a needy child. She was desperately insecure, yet she dressed in colours that seemed to exude self-confidence. The most striking thing about her, however, was her abnormally thin physique. She presented a picture of extreme malnourishment, yet she was just entering the 'blooming' stage of pregnancy. How was it possible for life to emerge in such conditions? I was reminded of those miraculous trees in the mountains which, against all the odds, burst into existence on sheer, barren rock faces. I congratulated her on the pregnancy and assured her of professional confidentiality.

"I have no secrets. Ask whatever you wish." She sat back in the chair, stroked the arm rests and fixed her eyes on me in anticipation of the first question. I started by asking her about her home life. She told me that she lived alone and had never been married.

"Is this your first pregnancy?"

"Sadly, yes. I always dreamed of having a family of my own but I've been far too busy attending to other people's needs. That's my lot in life, I guess. Don't get me wrong, I do it willingly, but it takes up a lot of time and energy, you know? My mother is completely reliant on me and one of my oldest friends has leukaemia so I'm constantly ferrying her to and from the hospital. It's impossible to find time for myself. I was resigned to the fact that I would never have a child and then quite unexpectedly, this!"

"You must be so excited. Are your friends and family supportive?"

"No one knows I'm pregnant," she said and then paused, perhaps remembering that only moments ago she had told me that she had no secrets.

"Oh. Why is that?"

"The father is one of my partners in the business."

"Have you told him?"

"I daren't. He'd be furious."

"Why would he be furious?"

"Because he already has five children. Because he won't leave his wife. Because he's monstrously selfish." She paused to draw breath and then launched into a catalogue of complaints about the man with whom she was going to have a child. Tor was one of three partners in a law firm specialising in asylum and human rights. After graduating from Oxford, she had volunteered in a Somali refugee camp before returning to London to study for her bar exams. She was a gifted orator whose eccentric manner and oddball humour rendered even the most mundane conversation entertaining. Her lover, whom she affectionately referred to as The Bastard, was ten years older than her, a bookish barrister with a booming voice and archaic manner. They had been conducting an affair for the past fifteen years and, unbeknownst to anyone, had bought an apartment together once the allure of hotels had worn off.

"Do you love this man?"

"It's not about love. It's convenient. It suits us both."

"Does he love you?"

"He's a married man! How can he love me? He's forever banging on about how miserable he is but he can't bring himself to leave his wife, despite the fact that he's been cheating on her for most of their marriage. He's obsessed with sex."

"Well, I guess that keeps things interesting!"

"We're not in our twenties, Gerad. Sometimes it's nice just to curl up on the sofa and talk, you know? I mean, he's not exactly a spring chicken." Tor was trying to elicit sympathy but her storytelling was so entertaining that I couldn't help but break into a smile. As I would come to discover, humour was one of many tools in her armoury, all of which were designed to draw the listener into her story of hardship and despair.

Early on in my training, the idea that you could make a diagnosis using nothing but the senses seemed absurd. It was said that JR Worsley could diagnose a patient's Causative Factor from the moment he walked into the room, using nothing but his sense of smell. It was a compelling story, but I had struggled to believe that it was actually true. However, slowly but surely, my scepticism had begun to wane. Walking into the student kitchen one afternoon, my nostrils began to sting with a putrid odour like that of urine. At precisely the same time, the woman making tea turned sharply to face me, a look of terror on her face. "Oh, it's you!" she said, before nonchalantly resuming her task. In that brief moment, I experienced two sensory signals – odour and emotion – as one, simultaneously alerting me to the Water element in distress. From that day onwards, I had wholeheartedly embraced the mystery of this system of medicine and endeavoured to master this unique method of diagnosis.

Tor and I had only spent a short time together, but I was already leaning heavily towards diagnosing the Earth element as the cause of her imbalance. Her odour was sickly sweet, and the pale yellow colour that fanned outwards from her temples was like that of an unripe fruit. Her voice, meanwhile, had an exaggerated, sing-song quality, and her incessant appeals for reassurance spoke of a desperate need to be understood. When the Earth element functions as Nature intended, it gives us the appetite to receive and savour everything that life offers. With our feet planted firmly on the ground, we feel self-assured, self-regulating and complete. My experience of Tor in those first few minutes told a very different story. Apparently devoid of that natural foundation, she seemed to be reaching out for the sustenance that she couldn't provide for herself. To test my assumptions, I decided to see how she would react if I offered her the sympathy she craved instead of engaging with her humour.

"Tor, it sounds like a really difficult and painful situation for you, so let's see if I can help you find a way through this." She sunk into her chair, a look of desperation etched across her face.

"You can't. It's hopeless. I knew it from the start but what else is there for me?" And with that she resumed the tirade against the man she loved to loathe, a quickfire volley of gripe and grievance. He was unkind to her, he criticised her appearance, he moaned about the mess in the flat. The unpacked boxes, the unhung pictures, the clothes on the floor, the dirty dishes. His driving was awful, his dress sense shocking, his personal hygiene prehistoric. She felt used by him, she couldn't bear it any longer. But what could she do? This push-pull dynamic was familiar to me. Sympathy is demanded but when it is offered it is immediately rejected, yet swiftly followed by the call for more. A look, a gesture, the apparent frustration of not being heard. It was like standing in front of an oscillating sphere, at once mesmerising and disorienting. I persevered, trying different ways to give her something to latch onto, but nothing landed.

One of the great joys of becoming a Five-Element acupuncturist is the knowledge gained through the study of Nature. Before learning about the Earth element, I took it for granted that I walked this planet with a sense of surety and stability. I never questioned how or why I could do this. This feeling of groundedness, even in the face of trouble, was a given for me. I vividly remember an elderly patient during the early years of my practice whom I had already diagnosed as having a Causative Factor in the Earth element before he told me that he felt as if he were living on a fault line. He described a constant state of dizziness that literally made him feel sick. He even walked with bowed legs, rocking from side to side as if to steady himself on the shifting ground beneath him. It wasn't until he had regained his equilibrium through treatment that he realised that what he was experiencing was anything but normal. It's exciting when I witness the Causative Factor manifesting in such a clear and unequivocal way, but the reality of practice is more nuanced, not least because the patient often exhibits numerous symptoms and behaviours that are unrelated to the Causative Factor.

'Heavenly Pivot' is an acupuncture point found on the Stomach channel just to the side of the navel. It is at our very centre, the place of perfect balance between Heaven above and Earth below. 'Heavenly Pivot' helps us to feel fully integrated in body, mind and spirit and provides us with a sense of security as we stand between these two great realms. However, it was clear to me that Tor would not yet be able to harness the full power of this point – there was still more foundational work to be done. Choosing acupuncture points is not a paint-by-numbers exercise. It is neither mechanical nor formulaic. On the contrary, the subtlety and efficacy of a treatment is entirely dependent on being able to sense what is happening with the patient in that precise moment. I felt that I needed more time to refine my diagnosis. 'Heavenly Pivot' would have to wait. It was time to switch gears.

"Tor, you've asked for my help but you don't seem willing to accept it. Tell me what I can do to help you change all this." She looked at me with a mixture of incomprehension and fury but stopped short of giving me an answer. It was clear that she didn't have one. Nor, I suspected, was she looking for one. Answers would deprive her of the only thing that she was familiar with: her misery. The cry for help was her raison d'être. God forbid that anyone should take that away from her.

"I do love him, but it's impossible. I desperately want the baby but…"

"But?"

"He won't agree to it. I'll have to get rid of it. If I don't, he'll leave me."

"Tor, I'm confused. You want me to help you with the pregnancy, yet you seem to feel that the whole situation is doomed. What is it that you really want from me?" She leaned forward, hung her head and fiddled with her hands. She had already begun telling herself that she couldn't have the child. Something would stand in the way. It always did.

"I don't know how to do it, Gerad."

"Do what, Tor?"

She stared at the ceiling for a moment as if the answer were up there somewhere, then slowly returned her gaze to the room and let out a long sigh. "Life! I don't know how to *do* life!"

I couldn't help but pause to consider the enormity of what she had just said. We all have our struggles but hers was all-encompassing, a fundamental inability to make sense of her existence or work out what she wanted from it. Tor was a highly accomplished lawyer, cultured, intelligent, witty and kind, but she was unable to derive satisfaction from anything. Everything was a problem by default. Worse still, any attempts to help her achieve the stability that she yearned for were met with resistance or outright rejection.

"Tor, let's step back and play with this for a moment. Let's imagine that you could get anything you want from these sessions. Anything at all. What would that be? What do you most want to change?"

"Change? You don't understand. This is the way it is for me. Nothing ever changes."

* * *

When I am with a patient, my primary focus is on making a diagnosis and constructing a treatment plan. It's tempting to slip into the psychotherapist's mindset, but raking over the coals of the past in search of answers, although helpful in building rapport, will not give me what I need to know. As much as I am engaged in a dialogue with my patients, their story doesn't help me to make a diagnosis. What matters is what's going on within. Fix that, and the story changes. What is the *cause* of a patient's symptoms or problems? I ask myself. The only way to answer that question is to pay attention to the senses and register what is inappropriate. A colour seen in the face that stands out from the complexion, a sound in the voice that grates on the ear, an inappropriate emotion that underpins everything they say and do, a disturbing odour that fills the room. Whatever is obviously out of kilter is what catches my attention. It is no different from hearing the distress in a friend's voice or seeing it in their demeanour. Somehow, you know that something is wrong.

I was now confident that Tor's Causative Factor was Earth. The first treatment was simple but powerful. I chose two of the acupuncture points known as the 'source points' – there are twelve of them in all, one on each of the meridians. Taoist philosophy teaches us that everything in the universe originates from one single source and that, in order to maintain the health of the whole, every part must remain connected to this source. By needling the source points, this treatment would provide the starting point for a return to balance and self-healing.

* * *

A week later, Tor returned. Our first meeting had been revealing in many ways, but it had also been perplexing. She had, after all, barely mentioned the pregnancy, the very thing that had supposedly motivated her to see me in the first place. What had become abundantly clear, however, was her pattern of behaviour. No matter what I said, it landed nowhere. If I agreed with her, she threw it back at me. If I sympathised with her, she scolded me for assuming I could understand. If I was kind to her, she was dismissive of my offer of warmth. Despite the unrelenting demand for sympathy, she was incapable of accepting it when it was offered. It was no wonder she couldn't stomach anything else in her life.

The beginning of the second session is always an edge-of-the-seat moment for the practitioner. The hope is that your patient will tell you that something has changed. A shift, a miracle, a revelation. The session began like the first one had – after twenty minutes she had barely drawn breath. She told me that since the previous week's treatment she had been suffering from migraines, nausea and chronic diarrhoea, all of which were described in vivid detail. It was the first time that any of these symptoms had appeared since her childhood. She had driven to the Welsh countryside to stay with friends but had spent the entire weekend slaving away in the kitchen while they were out enjoying the autumn sunshine. She felt neglected, taken for granted, used. One beef followed another before she turned her attention, as ever, to The Bastard, the hapless man who could do no right. Once again, the tongue-lashing was served up with relish, but then, all of a sudden, she stopped speaking and looked at me with a puzzled expression.

"Is there something else?"

"There is, yes. Even though the past week has been hellish, something feels different. It's difficult to explain but it's almost as if I noticed myself for the first time. The way I am, I mean. Does that sound weird?"

"Not at all. It's called waking up."

An unusual silence filled the room as she contemplated what I had said. "I looked at myself with disgust and I realised that I don't want to play this role any more. I don't want to be the schmuck that everyone takes advantage of."

"Is that really the way it is?"

"It's certainly what it feels like."

"But if it's just a role then you can change it, no?" Once again the prospect of a solution was too much for her and the moment of revelation was gone before it had a chance to take root. But something *had* changed. The first sign was the reappearance of historical symptoms, a classic example of the 'Law of Cure', which states that there is a tendency for things to get worse before they get better, but the bigger change was in her awareness of herself. She had, it seemed, had a glimpse of the person that she was before her tales of woe became her identity.

"Tor, have you thought about telling your partner that you're pregnant? Don't you think it would be better to start a dialogue sooner rather than later?"

"What's the point? There's no way he's going to let me keep it."

"Is that really so? Maybe he'll surprise you. Besides, isn't it ultimately your decision?"

Tor shook her head. "He's never going to give me what

I truly want." I waited for a moment to give her the chance to reflect on her words and then gestured for her to move to the treatment couch. It was September now, the season of the Earth element, when Nature is at her most abundant. When the harvest is finished, the farmers lay down their tools and gather together in the fields to appreciate the fruits of their labour. It's part of the natural cycle of life, yet it was something that Tor found herself unable to participate in. Despite all that she had achieved, she felt empty and insecure, so the focus of my treatment that day was twofold: firstly, in order to address this fundamental deficit within her, I chose two acupuncture points known as the 'horary points'. These points relate to the time of day and season, and would effectively reset her internal clock so that she would be aligned with the vibration and gifts of late summer. Secondly, I chose two points called the 'tonification points', which activate the creative cycle by stimulating the appetite of the Earth to draw energy from the Fire, just as a baby is drawn to suckle from its mother's breast. These points enact the immutable 'Law of Mother/Child', a force of Nature that drives creation, even in the harshest of circumstances.

* * *

A fortnight later, she was back.

"I told him."

"Well done. What was his reaction?"

"He said he was over the moon. He said he felt young again."

"That's wonderful, Tor. I'm so pleased for you."

"He's a barrister, Gerad. We're all actors in this profession."

I always looked forward to seeing Tor, but by the end of each session I was left feeling physically and emotionally drained. Not only was I beginning to understand her struggle intellectually, I was also being dragged into the weeds with her. In some ways she seemed more peaceful but, somewhere deep within, the innate capacity to feel fulfilled by her life experience lay dormant.

In the following weeks, the sessions followed a predictable pattern, with self-pitying stories delivered in such a captivating manner that I sometimes struggled to maintain my detachment. My role was to listen and, whenever there was a pause in the invective, offer a nod or a verbal affirmation that provided the fleeting fulfilment of her insatiable need for sympathy. Should I show even the slightest sign of disinterest, she would throw in her inimitable humour to give the gripe a softer edge and snag me once again. Many of us thrive on our problems because they legitimise our pleas for attention but, for most of us, there is eventually a resolution. In Tor's case, the lament was a powerful mental construct that never produced an outcome. The story was her identity and it could be boiled down to one sentence, one unrelenting appeal: "I need you to understand how I feel." Whenever there was a momentary lull, I tried a different line of enquiry to see if anything other than her energetic imbalance lay beneath the drama. How much of her story was actually real? I wondered. How much of it was a projection? And how much had she embellished it since she began telling it? It was so well crafted it was hard to imagine that this was its first rendition. On the contrary, it bore all the hallmarks of a carefully rehearsed, oft-repeated tale of misery.

In our next three sessions together, the treatments I gave Tor were designed to restore the power of the Stomach and the Spleen officials, whose strength, endurance and integrity would provide her with a strong foundation from which to navigate the shifting sands of her situation and sow the seeds of change. A sense of stability would help her stay grounded as she continued the process of healing, while a growing inner peace would enable her to acknowledge not only her weaknesses but also her strengths and how to use them to forge a path ahead. The 'spirit points' in Five-Element Acupuncture have beautiful names that describe the qualities that are seen in Nature and, when we are in balance, are reflected in each and every one of us. Each week I chose a combination of these powerful points. 'Receiving Fullness' gives us the capacity to absorb and appreciate the abundance and plenitude of the world around us. 'Leg Three Miles' gives us the wherewithal and resilience to stay the course. 'Earth Motivator' brings the possibility of radical change to body, mind and spirit. Just as the oxen turns the soil with the plough, so too would the rotovating action of this point help Tor to break down the relentless cycle of disappointment and prepare the ground for something new.

* * *

Lifelong patterns of behaviour are hard to break. Nevertheless, after our fifth session, the acupuncture treatments were still not producing the results that I would have expected, so at our next appointment, I decided that it was time to address the elephant in the room. Although she was abnormally underweight, Tor had always acted as if everything were entirely normal, conceding only that she needed to get back to the gym, so when she arrived on that day I was a little nervous. It was the first time that a patient of mine had made absolutely no mention of something that was so obviously contrary to her wellbeing. As soon as she arrived, she launched into her customary rant, but this time I stopped her in her tracks.

"Tor, you're now twenty-one weeks pregnant. Has your doctor talked to you about your body weight?" She pulled her shawl across her abdomen to conceal the bump and stared at me with barely concealed irritation.

"The baby is doing well. That's what he told me, anyway."

I persisted. "That's great but are *you* happy with your body weight?"

"What's happiness got to do with it? I eat like a horse but it goes right through me." I asked her about her daily food intake, and to my astonishment she described the diet of a wrestler, albeit a very picky one. "I'm permanently hungry. My friends think I'm anorexic but they don't understand." Tor had grown up in Portsmouth, one of five children. Her father was an engineer in the Royal Navy and was often at sea, so her mother effectively raised the family on her own. She was the middle child, the "pivot", as she put it. When I asked her what she meant, she said that she had to balance the family, to keep everything on an even keel. Shortly after her eleventh birthday, her father suddenly left. Her mother told her that he had gone to live with another woman. "That's when my weight plummeted. Before my father left, I was the fat girl but then… Well, something changed." Her mother was bemused. Tor started snacking between meals and binge eating during the night, yet within six months she had lost so much weight that she was diagnosed with an eating disorder. The doctor said it was bulimia but the diagnosis made no sense. Tor wasn't throwing up her food, she just couldn't digest it. Diarrhoea, or "the fat girl's friend", as she called it, was her constant companion. "The day my father left, it was as if he had reached inside and ripped out my centre. I was devastated. I no longer knew how to be in this world. That feeling has never gone away."

"Did your mother comfort you?"

"She didn't have time for me. She had the twins to care for, so I had to fend for myself."

After her father's departure, Tor had also started to develop symptoms of obsessive compulsive disorder, constantly checking that all of the windows in the house were closed and laying the table over and over again to ensure that everything was in perfect symmetry. Then the restless nights began. At the foot of her bed was an antique chest that she would open and close periodically throughout the night.

"I couldn't get the thought out of my head that there might be something inside," she told me. "I was convinced that if I didn't get out of bed and check, I would die in my sleep." This lonely obsession consumed her for almost two years.

"Your father, is he still in your life?"

"Good God, no. Why would I let him into my life? We weren't good enough for him, so I'm not going to crawl back to him and make him feel OK about destroying our family. What is it with men? Do they have no idea what it feels like to be abandoned?" And then, as quickly as she had become irritated, her expression softened and she broke into a generous smile. "Shall we get our next session in the diary? I do like having something to look forward to." She reached for her Filofax and began leafing through the pages. "Next week is pretty horrendous but maybe Tuesday? No, Tuesday is impossible. Wednesday? I'm having lunch with that dreadful woman at the Home Office and then I'm at the Refugee Council for most of the afternoon. Maybe sometime after seven? You don't mind staying a bit later than usual, do you? I like coming at the end of the day in case we need more time together."

* * *

A week later, Tor arrived late for her appointment. She looked different as she sat in the chair. Her body language was submissive and there was a palpable silence.

"Are you OK, Tor?" I asked. The look in her eyes was one of utter defeat.

"I got rid of it. My baby. I terminated the pregnancy." I was stunned. I leaned forward to take her hand but she pulled away, folded her arms in a gesture of defiance and threw her head back to stop the tears. I was lost for words. To have conceived at her age and in her condition had been nothing short of miraculous. To have ended the pregnancy at twenty-three weeks was not only unbearably sad but also shocking. "I desperately wanted a child but I was convinced he didn't want me to have it. I thought he would leave me. What could I do?"

"I'm so sorry, Tor." She shuffled awkwardly in the chair.

"I didn't believe him. I couldn't."

"Have you told him?"

"Yes." She paused, visibly upset. "He was mad with rage. He said I had murdered our child. He said I was mentally unfit to be a mother or a partner." For a moment the only sound in the room was the ticking of the clock and the rustling of leaves coming from the open window that gave onto the gardens above. I thought of the terrible impact that those words must have had and the unimaginable pain of having aborted her child.

"What will you do now?"

"There's nothing to do. It's over. He left me."

* * *

Tor stopped coming for treatment. I wrote several times to ask how she was but my messages went unanswered, which I found troubling. As much as I try to maintain a degree of detachment from my patients' lives, it isn't always possible and in this instance I had a nagging sense of personal responsibility. Had I somehow been complicit? Had my diagnosis been correct? Had I chosen the right points? Had I supported her enough? These thoughts consumed me and challenged everything I had learned about being the 'instrument' while at the same time giving love to my patients. I sought advice from a colleague, who patiently listened as I recounted the case history, and then reassured me that my approach had been correct.

Two years passed, and then one day, I heard a familiar voice on my voicemail.

"Gerad, I walked past your clinic yesterday. Your petunias need watering."

A week later, Tor was sitting cross-legged in the armchair opposite me, launching into an animated tirade about everything and everyone. Noisy neighbours, the government, the pigeons on her roof, the pictures in the waiting room. And then, almost as an afterthought, she told me why she had come.

"We're back together. Me and The Bastard. We've decided to try for a child again. We're using donor eggs this time. My doctor told me that I need to put on weight. I thought perhaps you could help me."

"Of course, I have complete faith in you. I'll do whatever I can to help." Tor seemed to bask in my words of encouragement, but as I watched this formidable woman in her habitual posture, gently caressing the patches of soft worn leather on the arms of the chair, she suddenly seemed very small and vulnerable. I marvelled at her tenacity and resilience, but at the same time I was worried for her. Was she once again mistaking the illusion of home and family for the inner stability that she unconsciously yearned for? And what about me? Was I on the right track? Had I adopted the best treatment strategy to help her? We talked for a while and it was apparent that little had changed. She still had a voracious appetite, yet she looked weary and weak. Her friends, her family, her lover, her life, everything was a bitter disappointment. Even her work, which she spoke of with such pride, left her feeling despondent. She was, quite simply, unable to digest anything. And so, rather than embark on yet another cycle of sympathy and rejection, I decided to take a different approach.

"Tor, to support the acupuncture treatment I want you to make some changes that should help you to achieve a better outcome. First of all, can we agree that you're not that great at looking after yourself?" She nodded. "OK, so it's time to change that. You need to start giving yourself what you need, and don't assume that because you are forty-six years old you know what that is. Very few people do. Be gentle and kind with yourself. From now on, at any given moment, get into the habit of asking yourself: 'What is it that I need? Am I hungry? Am I thirsty? Am I lonely? Am I tired?' And then respond to those needs as a mother would to a child."

"Asking myself what I need sounds simple enough. But what if I don't know?"

"We'll work it out together." I expected a rebuttal yet, to my surprise, she became quite animated with excitement. I felt as if I had been given a second chance to help her, and so I vowed not to get caught up in her story if I could possibly help it. Instead, I would focus my attention relentlessly on the sensory signals in front of me, just as I had been taught. I reminded myself that the unfolding of another person's life is neither my business nor my responsibility. My role is to listen to what Nature is asking me to do to assist this miraculous process.

Tor came for weekly treatment and she thrived. One of the most obvious signs of change was the feel of her hands. Several times during a treatment, I take the patient's hands in mine and place my fingertips over the radial pulse to read the balance and flow of energy. It is often a very telling moment. When Tor first came to see me, her hand was sticky and tense. Now it was warm, dry and relaxed, a clear sign of a more confident and settled inner state. A month later, two embryos were transferred and she became pregnant with twins. At six weeks there were two heartbeats, at ten weeks the embryos were the perfect size and at twelve weeks everything was proceeding exactly as it should. Then, fourteen weeks into the pregnancy, she came to see me.

"The twins," she said. "They're gone. I miscarried them both." I leaned forward to take her hand and this time there was no resistance. She lowered her head and then, for the first time since we had met, we sat together in silence. I thought back to our first encounter, the day that this vivacious, larger-than-life character had appeared in my waiting room, cup in hand, and invited me into her world. In many ways she had improved. Despite the apparent turmoil of her outer life, she had begun to establish a greater sense of peace within – but each time she was knocked by a new drama, the self-defeating thoughts and behaviour returned. Deep down, she was still unable to abandon her belief that life was unfair, and this latest devastating blow only served to confirm this compelling narrative in her mind. She had, she said, hit a new low. Indeed, she looked broken.

Many years ago, I called an old and trusted friend, a highly respected psychotherapist, and asked her if I could refer a patient of mine to her. The man in question was a chronic alcoholic whose life was falling apart. She asked me to describe his situation, but when I had finished she said, "He's not ready. Let me know when he's hit rock bottom, then I'll see him." Destructive patterns of behaviour repeat themselves until they are broken, sometimes by sheer force of will but more often than not by some cataclysmic event. For most of us, it is only when everything has come crashing down that we are finally able to forge a different path. Until now, Tor had been stuck in an endless cycle of dissatisfaction, desperately trying to soothe the overwhelming feeling of discontent by changing the outer conditions of her life instead of looking within. If only she could have a child, if only her lover would leave his wife, if only people wouldn't take her for granted, then everything would be OK. Now, finally, the illusion had shattered. The stories wouldn't work any more. She had reached rock bottom.

"I think we have some more work to do, Tor." She looked up at me, wiped the tears from her eyes and silently nodded her acquiescence.

BROKEN BOWL

* * *

Like many of us, Tor had been scarred by her childhood, but it was not so much the circumstances of her younger years that had shaped her adulthood as her inherent inability to embrace and contain the richness of day-to-day life. The ancient Chinese cultivated this skill by observing and experiencing the gifts of each season. Late summer and the Earth element give us the capacity to layer the wealth of our life experiences, good and bad, in order to create inner strength, stability and abundance. Without this capacity, life's gifts pass through us like water from a broken bowl, and with them the promise of contentment. Our behaviour and the choices we make lead us inexorably towards a life of disappointment and despair.

In my line of work, breakthroughs are gradual. Sure, there are moments of enlightenment, but generally the improvements are incremental. The chaos on the outside and the peace within are like parallel lines that gradually converge as awareness grows and balance is restored, but it is an ongoing process. Awareness is not an end in itself. Rather, it gives us the ability to observe the inevitable ups and downs of life and treat them with equanimity. As the weeks passed, Tor slowly began to understand that she could have a harmonious relationship with life and leave behind the feeling of ungroundedness that had troubled her for so long. The belief that she could never have what she wanted started to subside and the need to constantly seek the attention and sympathy of others began to lose its former strength. Her colour and the sound of her voice changed, as did her odour. Even her wardrobe changed, the garish colours replaced by more subtle shades that spoke of a growing self-assurance.

In the months following the miscarriage, the process of real recovery accelerated. Tor committed herself to a programme of self-care, and the acupuncture treatments began to bear fruit in a most unexpected way. While it didn't altogether disappear, her reflexive tendency to blame others and bathe in self-pity became an object for exploration as she learned to take responsibility for herself. As part of this natural process of self-healing, she revisited the termination of her pregnancy, acknowledging the intense pain she felt, while allowing herself the depth of self-forgiveness and compassion needed to transcend the memory of that traumatic event. She was stronger in every way and, when she spoke, she did so with measured eloquence and poignancy, without losing her inimitable wit. It was as if she was ripening from the centre. Two of my favourite points – 'Abundant Splendour' and 'Prince's Grandson' – whetted Tor's appetite for the richness and magic of life, while 'Great Enveloping' gave her the capacity to both fully embrace her new-found freedom and feel securely wrapped in the arms of life itself. By modelling a genuine compassion and empathy for her, I helped her to find these same qualities within herself, just as a mother teaches a baby the art of self-soothing. As she began to establish a solid emotional bedrock, her behaviour and her choices started to change. She ended her seventeen-year affair and relinquished her partnership at the law firm to commence training as a counsellor for refugees. She also put on a little weight and started a new relationship with an academic in his sixties.

"What's his name?" I asked when we next met.

She grinned mischievously. "Sugar Daddy."

"Perfect! Better a sugar daddy than a bastard, right?"

"Absolutely. I did well, didn't I?"

When I last saw her, Tor told me that she and her Sugar Daddy were considering adoption. The memory of the termination continued to plague her, but the way that she had reframed her story, together with a new-found inner stability, enabled her to look back on her life with a level of self-compassion and acceptance that was previously unimaginable.

2

ILLUMINATED SEA

*

Dylan sat bolt upright in his chair, his eyes scanning the room. He was dressed in a brown blazer, light blue jumper and ill-fitting grey trousers that revealed patterned ankle socks and a pair of weathered brogues, one of which was beginning to come away from its sole. In his left hand, he was holding a scrap of paper covered in handwritten notes.

"Can I get you some water?" I asked. He looked startled. "Er, no thanks." I was already starting to feel uneasy around my new patient, but what struck me most of all was the smell of wet dog, an odour so intense that it had filled the room. Catching a hint of this would normally provide me with one of the four legs of the stool that I need to make a diagnosis, but this was off the scale. Could it really be coming from the man sitting opposite me? Or was it his jacket, an old waxed Barbour that had clearly seen better days? There was only one way to find out.

"Can I take your coat for you?" Dylan removed the oily Barbour without budging from the chair and held it out for me. I got to my feet, hung the jacket on the back of the door and returned to my seat. The stagnant odour still hung in the air but it was clearly not coming from the coat, which was now at the far end of the room. It had to be my patient. Assuming my sense of smell was not deceiving me, the first leg of the stool was in place.

Dylan was an unsmiling man in his late thirties with long, taut limbs and feet that turned inwards. His eyes were the colour of obsidian, ringed with dark circles. What struck me most from a diagnostic perspective, however, was the colour around his temples: a subtle diffusion of blue, like the remnants of a dye that had long ago soaked into his pale, blotchy skin. He looked as if he had just crawled out from under a rock. And he looked terrified.

"Why do you have a clipboard? Are you going to take notes?"

"Don't worry, I write very little down. Just enough to jog my memory."

He stared at me without a flicker of emotion and then inhaled sharply. "I damage cars," he announced. "I can't stop…" He paused, perhaps waiting for a reaction, but I said nothing. "It started when I was a kid… I got into a fight with my dad and I went to my room and drank a load of vodka and then I walked into the village and there was an old Rolls Royce parked in the lane in front of the church and… I don't know what made me do it but I scratched it all the way down the side with my house key." He suddenly dried up and locked eyes with me, but it was not an invitation to join the conversation. Apparently, he just needed a moment to refuel, because before I could say anything he was off again, a look of panic etched across his face. "That was a long time ago but I still do it… I don't know why… After work sometimes I walk across the bridge to Westminster and when the coast is clear I pick out a car and then… I walk past and drag a key down the side… It's an amazing feeling." Dylan's gaze had become distant as he described this strange obsession, but he came back to the room with a jolt and his eyes narrowed. "If you tell anyone I'll lose my job."

I was so taken aback by this garbled confession that I was momentarily lost for words. I was also feeling distinctly unsettled, not so much by what he had told me, but the way in which he had recounted it. He would stutter and stumble as if he were too nervous to continue, but then his thoughts would come gushing out in a deluge of words. Listening to him grated on me, but for most of the session, listening was all I could do because the chances to interrupt were few and far between.

"OK, Dylan, let's rewind for a second. I appreciate your willingness to open up to me, but we've got plenty of time."

He looked taken aback. "Did I say something wrong?"

"Not at all, but I'd like to hear a bit more about you and your background first, and then we can talk in more detail about why you came to see me. We'll work this out together, OK?"

Over the next twenty minutes or so, I began to get a sense of Dylan's life and what had motivated him to seek my help. What was abundantly clear from the start was that he needed a reassuring presence in the room. Even the slightest unexpected sound or movement sent him into a panic, so I stayed absolutely still and allowed him to offload. Once he felt safe in my presence, the intensity of his odour began to dissipate, his speech returned to a more measured rhythm and, slowly but surely, he started to open up. Dylan had grown up in a small village in Sussex, the son of a Welshman who ran the local pub. His mother died when he was sixteen and his father remarried within a matter of months. Dylan hid away in his room.

"I spent hours every day listening to music through my headphones so I could shut out all the noise from downstairs… I used to compose stuff, too."

Generally speaking, leading questions are counter-productive because they buy into the idea that I can somehow make a diagnosis from the story of someone's life. Nevertheless, I was curious to know if this desire to withdraw was a reaction to his mother's death or a repeating pattern throughout his childhood.

"Did you always like to spend time on your own?"

"Yeah, my dad tried to get me involved with the pub but the whole thing made me really uncomfortable so I spent most of the time upstairs with my dog."

Dylan's father was from Cardiff, but he had lived in Portsmouth until the break-up of his first marriage. He had been in the navy but retired early for reasons that were not entirely clear. The official story was that he had been injured but Dylan suspected it had something to do with his shore leave antics.

"Let's just say that my dad likes to have a good time… He's a decent fella but we're like chalk and cheese… I guess he couldn't understand how he ended up with a son who wasn't interested in rugby and women and all that stuff, so after mum was diagnosed with cancer, I kept myself to myself."

"I imagine your mother's illness must have been very difficult for you."

Dylan tensed his shoulders. "Not at all. We're all going to die, right?" His response sounded nonchalant, coldhearted even, but my senses told me something different. His odour and the blue colour around his temples, both of which had suddenly intensified, were a clear indication that he was not OK.

"What was your childhood like? Before your mother died, I mean."

"There wasn't much to do in the village but I was good with computers, so I taught myself to code, and there was a maths club in Eastbourne that I used to go to quite often. Anything to escape."

Before I knew it he was in full flow again, a grinding monologue about village life, the suffocating sea mist and the graffiti-strewn shelter where he waited for the bus to Eastbourne. He talked about the pub, how he used to look for loose change under the seat cushions, and how he had enough money to buy a keyboard by the time he was seventeen. Saving money was important, he told me. There was no telling what the future might bring. Staying tuned into what he was saying was a challenge, not because it was uninteresting but because once again it was delivered in a persistent, monotonous groan. Yet as much as it jangled my nerves, the sound of his voice was also a gift. I already had the odour and the colour. Now, it seemed, I had the sound. Unless I was very much mistaken, this was the third leg of the stool.

Had I met Dylan before I became an acupuncturist, I would almost certainly have written him off as a rather tiresome man, but learning how the five elements shape and inform our reality has fundamentally changed the nature of my interaction with everyone I encounter. The behavioural oddities that once would have set me on edge are now a source of fascination. People still drive me mad occasionally, but nowadays I view human behaviour through a different lens, one that blows my mind. I can literally see the five elements having a meltdown in front of my eyes.

Dylan's monologue continued but then, all of a sudden, the words petered out. I seized the opportunity to interrupt before he had a chance to recover.

"Were you happy as a kid?"

Dylan looked panicked. "I dunno. Maybe? I just… I just felt very uncomfortable a lot of the time."

"What do you mean by uncomfortable?"

"I found it hard to get involved in anything… Everyone else at school was much more chilled. Same thing at home… My parents wanted me to mix with the other kids in the village, but I felt like a fish out of water, so I did my own thing."

"Did you have friends?"

"Just one, a girl called Rachel, the daughter of my music teacher… We're still close… She used to do the vocals for some of my compositions… She was the one who introduced me to free climbing. We used to go to the South Downs and climb up these crazy rock faces without ropes or anything."

"It sounds terrifying."

"Nah, not at all. I love it. It's a place I feel really comfortable... I'll never forget the first time I was up there on the rock face... It's hard to describe, but it was like an out-of-body experience... The more dangerous it was, the better I felt."

"Adrenaline. Best drug in town."

"I hadn't thought of it like that." Dylan had become visibly calm as he recalled the climbing, but when my phone suddenly rang he almost jumped out of his skin.

"I'm so sorry, Dylan." I quickly turned it off but he was clearly rattled. It was intriguing to see how easily he was knocked off balance and how long it took him to settle again. But what struck me most of all was that no matter what we talked about, there was a constant undertow of fear. It had been apparent from the moment he walked into my room and it spoke volumes. Could this be the final leg of the stool? Making a diagnosis is often challenging but occasionally the sensory signals that point to the cause of imbalance seem almost impatient to reveal themselves. Dylan was one such case, perhaps because he was so completely out of kilter. His body, mind and spirit had become stagnant and polluted, and they were crying out for help. The blue around the temples, the unrelenting groan, the putrid odour and the tangible feeling of fear: all four sensory signals were leading me inexorably towards the murky, mysterious world of the Water element with its associated officials, the Bladder and the Kidney.

"OK, Dylan, I've got what I need. I'm going to wash my hands and then I'd like to see what's going on with you. Shoes and socks off, please, then make yourself comfortable on the treatment couch." When I came back into the room, Dylan was lying completely still, his eyes fixed on the ceiling, his arms stuck rigidly to his sides. I took his left hand and placed it in mine. I was curious to see if he would relax, even a little, but he gripped my hand like a drowning man hanging on for dear life. I closed my eyes and began to feel the twelve Chinese pulses. Superficial, deep, superficial, deep, superficial, deep. I released his hand and moved round to the other side of the couch, his eyes tracking my every step. I picked up his right hand and placed my fingers on his wrist. Superficial, deep, superficial, deep, superficial, deep. I let go of his hand and walked over to my desk to make a note of the readings, but no sooner had I picked up my pen than I heard his panicked voice.

"Is everything OK?"

Dylan's nervous energy was unsettling and, as often happens, it began to rub off on me. After thirty years of practice, I am very confident of my clinical skills, but all of a sudden I found myself fumbling around like a novice, dropping the needles and questioning my ability to locate the acupuncture points. If I hadn't figured out by now that this patient operated from fear, the way that I was spontaneously reacting to him would have told me so.

I kept the first treatment simple but powerful: two bilateral points that support the Water element by re-establishing the connection of its officials – the Bladder and Kidney – to the source. According to the Chinese classics, Water "holds the memory of the Divine". In other words, this baseline element contains the blueprint from which all life emerges. If my diagnosis was correct and the Water element was indeed the underlying cause of Dylan's imbalance, then this intervention with my needles would immediately create a change in all twelve officials and their related pulses. By the end of the treatment, Dylan looked peaceful. A sense of calm had returned to the room and the smell of stagnant water had all but gone. I was clearly on the right track.

* * *

My first session with Dylan had been somewhat intense; however, despite the drama, it was clear to me that what he was struggling with was the outcome not only of his personal history but rather a heightened level of fear that, unbeknownst to him, drove everything that he thought, said and did. When we lose our way in life, the tendency is to project what we feel inside onto the world around us, instead of looking within and taking responsibility for those feelings. Dylan was no exception. Deprived of the natural capacity to find the reassurance that the Water element gives us, he perceived the world as a fearful place over which he sought to assert his control. As it turned out, his initial confession was just a taste of things to come, for bubbling under the surface of this highly driven man was a catalogue of long-suppressed secrets that seemed to fuel his sense of dread. First, he had tested the waters, but once the floodgates had been opened, it all came pouring out.

Our second meeting was on a cold day in December. As I walked into the reception area, Eszter caught my eye and twisted her face into an expression of wide-eyed terror.

"Your patient is here."

I smiled and gave her an appreciative nod. "Thank you, Eszter." The waiting room was full of hunched figures tapping on their smartphones. In the far corner, I could just make out Dylan's face, half submerged beneath the folds of a large scarf. He was wearing a pair of oversized headphones and his eyes were sweeping the room like searchlights. As soon as he spotted me, he leapt to his feet with a startled look, removed the headphones and approached me with an outstretched hand that was cold and damp to the touch. I led him down the narrow stairs and into my treatment room. He sat down without taking his jacket off and placed his scarf and notebook on his knees.

"Welcome back, Dylan. How are you doing?"

"Pretty good, actually. Remarkably good, in fact. I've felt lighter, happier even."

"That's good to hear. Have you noticed anything in particular?"

"Well, for starters I haven't scratched a single car. I felt the urge but… Well, what can I say? I didn't."

Compared to our first meeting, Dylan seemed calm and composed. He still had the look of someone who had just seen a ghost but he was altogether warmer and more engaging. Perhaps most notably of all, his odour had changed. For the better.

"How has your sleep been?"

"I've been going to bed early and sleeping through till six. That's never happened before."

"Even when you were young?"

"Especially when I was young." As a child, Dylan had attended the local comprehensive school but, like so many kids, he had more or less been written off after being diagnosed with Attention Deficit Hyperactivity Disorder (ADHD). "They had no concept of how to deal with someone like me. The doctor prescribed Ritalin, which kind of worked, but my music teacher is the one I really have to thank. She took me under her wing. My maths teacher, too. If it wasn't for them, I don't know what would have become of me." With the help of his mentors, Dylan had defied all expectations, year after year. By the time he was eighteen he had received an offer from Imperial College to study Computer Science. "Artificial intelligence and machine learning was my thing. Anthropology for robots." He let slip a rare smile but quickly retreated to the safety of his wary demeanour.

"So you moved to London?"

"No, no. I lived at home until I graduated. I used to take the train in from Brighton."

"No social life, then?"

"No time for that. I was there to learn."

"Girlfriends?" Silence. "Boyfriends?"

"No!"

It was no surprise to hear that Dylan was gifted. His presence in the treatment room was intense and it was clear that his somewhat subdued presence and stuttering manner belied a towering intellect. Despite my wobble during the first treatment, being with him brought out the best in me. Everything I did was closely watched, so there was no room for error.

In his final year, just as he was beginning to look for opportunities in the private sector, Dylan was approached by the intelligence services.

"MI6. I didn't see that one coming but it's great. I got lucky."

"What is it that you like most about it?"

"The security." I smiled but his stony face told me that it was an unintentional pun.

"You mean the pension?"

"Exactly. But it's not just that. I'm in my element there. It's a natural fit."

I knew better than to ask any more. In thirty years, I've only ever had one patient who wasn't allowed to talk about his job and that was Dylan. To this day, I have no idea if he was hacking into the Kremlin's mainframe or sweeping floors. In some ways it felt as though I was missing something, such is the importance that we put on our professional identity, yet somehow it was appropriate for a man who gave so little away. From his job to his personal relationships, his life seemed to have a continuous thread of secrecy running through it. The self-imposed isolation, the furtive acts of petty vandalism, the mystery surrounding his sexual orientation. All of it was hidden away, blanketed in fear, never to be spoken of.

To the casual observer, Dylan might have seemed rather dull and colourless. He might also have come across as rather tedious. Yet beneath the surface of this mysterious, tortured man was an intense power yet to be realised. The Water element gives us the ability and drive to be our authentic self. When it is out of balance, we feel inert, lifeless even. When it functions as it should, we emerge from the depths of our being, innately aware of our potential, and grow effortlessly into an uncompromising expression of ourselves. My treatment strategy for Dylan was to help him reawaken his inner power and harness it in a way that would allow him to step comfortably into his true self. To move, in other words, from surviving to thriving.

I allowed the conversation to go on longer than usual that day, relishing the relative ease of the exchange, but I had been lulled into a false sense of security. Never turn your back to the ocean, as they say. Just when you think the water is calm, a wave appears out of nowhere and knocks you to the ground. Thirty minutes into the session, I brought the conversation to a close and was about to get to my feet to prepare for the treatment when Dylan stopped me.

"Wait," he said. "There's something else…" He shuffled uneasily in his chair. "There's something else I need to tell you." I nodded and waited for him to continue. "You know I told you… the Ritalin… you know I told you about the Ritalin?"

"Yes, you take it for the ADHD, right?"

Dylan shook his head. "I take it, but not for the ADHD."

"I'm not sure I understand."

"The thing is, I… I hoard it… and… and then…" Dylan stopped and stared at me, seemingly unable to get his words out. "You see, I'm supposed to take it every morning but I don't… I save it up and then I binge on it… Every few weeks, I binge on it."

"How much do you take?"

"A lot… I stay up all night… All weekend sometimes… I watch porn… I binge on it and watch porn." The discovery of Dylan's private life felt significant. Until then he had studiously avoided any discussion of his sexuality, and whatever desires he may have had seemed to have been suppressed. Now, all of a sudden, he had admitted to having a sexual appetite, albeit a somewhat unconventional one. Most people express their sexuality effortlessly, but for Dylan, the idea of making himself look attractive or flirting were completely alien. The absence of social interaction and the expression of his sexual energy through the use of medication and pornography were yet more evidence of the troubling secrets that lay hidden beneath the exterior of this seemingly unremarkable man.

Dylan's revelations brought to mind something I had learned early on in my studies. The main trunk of the body is divided into three sections – lower, middle and upper – which are called the "three burning spaces". The lower section, located below the navel, is the designated home of the Water element and is likened in the classical texts to a swamp or a ditch. It has the feeling of a dark underworld: cold, mysterious and full of potential. As Dylan spoke that day, it felt as if the swamp was slowly beginning to release its secrets. My hope was that it would also begin to release its power. As compelling as peoples' stories can be, my role in the treatment room is to respond to Nature's alarm bells and design a treatment that will bring my patient back to balance. Dylan's tale was fascinating and I have no doubt that a psychoanalyst would have had a field day trying to work out the reasons for his behaviour, but for me it was simple. Nature had provided me with clear sensory signals that had pointed me in the direction of the Water element. It's important to remember that our bodies are sixty per cent water, so it's not surprising that this element needs to be carefully managed at all times. The Chinese character for 'water' is also used to signify 'power' and 'flow', both of which are essential for the maintenance of life. In Dylan's case, these qualities were chaotic and inconsistent, giving rise to all manner of symptoms and inappropriate behaviour.

'Bubbling Spring' is the first point on the Kidney meridian and its function is to unleash our innate strength and potential. It is likened to the purest water that rises from the earth at the source of a river, high up in the mountains. As it carves a path through the valleys and winds its way across the plains, it brings life to everything. 'Great Brightness' is a point found on a section of the Kidney meridian that passes through the lower abdomen (the dark swamp). It brings warmth and light to the region to illuminate the depths of who we are. 'Fly and Scatter', a point on the Bladder meridian, helps to release the deep reservoirs of energy that will drive us forward and enable us to enter fully into life. As the treatments progressed, Dylan's cold and suspicious presence gradually gave way to a warmer and friendlier being and his tendency to withdraw, driven by the need to protect his depleted reserves of energy, began to subside. Little by little, he became aware of a growing inner drive to fulfil his destiny.

* * *

Dylan came to see me every week like clockwork, and each time he prepared for the session in meticulous detail, writing down everything he wanted to say so he wouldn't forget anything. He was always courteous, but it was obvious that developing a more intimate relationship with me was not on his agenda. The week after telling me about the Ritalin binges, he reported feeling much better.

"I don't know what you did with those needles but it's powerful stuff. I feel so much calmer and energised."

"Calmer? In what way?"

"In the way I am. I've always been driven to succeed but I hadn't realised how anxious and obsessive I can be. I'm starting to see that now. I decided to knock the Ritalin on the head. I haven't touched it. It wasn't easy but it feels liberating."

Coming off medication was a big step and it was one that he had apparently taken without any help. My worry was that it wouldn't endure; that the sudden withdrawal would precipitate a crisis. I suggested that he let his doctor know that he was no longer taking the prescribed medication and then I held out my hand to congratulate him.

"It's not easy to tackle compulsions, especially if you're not even aware of them."

He gripped my hand tightly and smiled. "That's it, isn't it? I've been on autopilot. It never occurred to me to step back and look at what I was doing."

"First comes awareness, then comes change."

"The Buddha?"

"Confucius." Offering pearls of ancient wisdom to my patients generally evokes a positive reaction. With Dylan, however, it was like tossing pebbles into a pond. There was a momentary acknowledgement of the gift, a ripple on the surface of the water, but it would always take time to sink in. "Tell me, is there anything going on at the moment that might disturb this peace that you've found?"

"The thing that's really bugging me at the moment is my job… I love it, but the woman I report to is making my life hell. I don't understand it because I'm pretty good at what I do, but she seems determined to undermine me."

"In what way?"

"Putting me down, diminishing my achievements… I don't know what her motivation is but it's really getting me down. One minute she's all smiles and the next thing I know she's having a go at me…"

"Why don't you say something?"

"There's no point. It won't make any difference."

"But don't you think it's important for her to know that her actions are upsetting you?"

"She already knows that. That's why she does it."
"Can't you talk to someone higher up the chain?"
"I don't want to rock the boat."

Despite having asked for my help, nothing I suggested made a difference. For Dylan, the idea of confrontation was intensely uncomfortable, and his reluctance to face up to challenging situations meant that the emotions they provoked remained buried. The tension built and built until it could no longer be contained and eventually he was compelled to release it in altogether unhealthy ways.

The focus of my treatment didn't change. My principal objective was to restore the healthy functioning of the Bladder and Kidney officials. These two organs work on a physiological level, in that they govern the reservoirs and flow of water through the body, but they also work on the mind and spirit. 'Greater Mountain Stream' on the Kidney channel is likened to the freshness and strength of a river as it flows with gathering strength through creeks and gorges. The Bladder Official is responsible for the so-called 'cultivation of yin' the earliest stage of manifestation, which is likened to the formation of our skeleton – the deepest part of ourselves. According to the classics, the journey of its meridian lays out the "regions and territories", an epic unfolding of our entire being. 'Golden Gate', the sixty-third of sixty-seven points on the Bladder channel, gives us the reassuring feeling that the journey is almost complete, the final gate through which we pass before arriving at the 'Extremity of Yin'. Together, these two points help the Bladder and the Kidney rediscover their unique roles and, in turn, the Water element builds

THE UNTAPPED SELF

in strength by harnessing its own inherent power.

A week later, Dylan was back, but my hope that he would have found the courage to deal with the situation was quickly dashed. "I've asked for a transfer," he told me. "I can't take it any more. A few days ago she told me that my personal hygiene was an issue. She said I should consider using deodorant."

"Seriously? How did you react when she said that to you?"

"I told her that I take a shower every morning. What else could I say?"

"And you would rather move to another department than deal with the situation?"

Dylan froze like a deer in the headlights. "I'm loath to move. I've worked hard to get where I am but I just don't have it in me to work with people like that. I'll be OK."

* * *

Two months had passed since Dylan had first come to see me. He had made considerable progress, but I still had the sense that something was getting in the way. One day in late April, he was due for an early morning appointment but turned up late. He was flustered and his speech was once again rushed and rambling.

"You seem troubled, Dylan. Are you OK?"

"Everything's OK, it's OK…" I remained still and waited for him to continue. "Look, something happened many years ago but it's OK… Actually it's not OK, there's something else I need to tell you." Dylan removed his jumper and placed it on the floor beside his chair. He started to say something and then stopped abruptly. He was clenching his fists repeatedly as if he were trying to squeeze the tension out.

"What is it, Dylan? It's OK, you can tell me. I'm here to help you, not judge you."

"Something bad happened… It… it was a long time ago but I'm terrified that it's going to come out. I can't stop thinking about it, I can't sleep, it's like everything's been stirred up, everything from the past. I thought I'd put it behind me."

When Dylan was sixteen, he and his father had spent Christmas with their cousins in Wales. His aunt and uncle had a big house that backed onto a forest, where Dylan and his cousin, Rhys, walked the dogs and collected kindling for the fire.

"It was a really cold Christmas that year, I remember it clearly. My dog kept on disappearing into the snow drifts. Me and Rhys, we used to walk for hours. He was quite a bit younger than me but he was a really bright kid. One day we were talking… about stuff… I asked him if he masturbated… He said he didn't know much about anything like that. We were sharing a room and that night I told him I would teach him how to do it. I thought he wouldn't say anything, I mean I was just… I was just showing him, but he must have told his mother. A few months later, she came to see my dad and accused me of being a pervert… I could hear them talking about it and my dad… he was trying to play the whole thing down and…"

"Did your father talk to you about it?"

"He never mentioned it, not a word... But ever since then I've lived in fear of it coming out. It'd destroy me."

When Dylan stopped speaking the silence in the room was palpable. He sat perfectly still but his eyes betrayed the feeling of dread that was consuming him from within. His addictions, his guilt, his paranoia, his shame. Little by little, all of his fears were beginning to overwhelm him.

* * *

The process of healing is different for everyone and it rarely happens in a linear fashion. Many of my patients come with the expectation that they will see tangible improvements after each treatment, but that's not necessarily the way Nature works. If they are treated directly, some symptoms may be quick to disappear, but there is no telling when other more profound problems, many of them long forgotten or wilfully repressed, will rise to the surface. One thing is for sure, though: if the underlying cause is treated, they will. And when they do, they tend to manifest in unexpected ways. In Dylan's case, it was particularly dramatic.

A few weeks later, he didn't show up for his appointment. I called and left messages on his phone but he didn't reply. The following evening, just as my final patient of the day was leaving, the buzzer went. I double-checked my diary but nobody was booked in, so I walked upstairs to see who was waiting for me. I was met at the top of the stairs by Eszter, who was frowning.

"There's a woman here to see you. I told her she needed to make an appointment but she said it couldn't wait." I walked into the waiting room to find a woman in her mid-thirties dressed from top to bottom in dark denim. She stood up and greeted me warmly. "I'm so pleased to meet you, Gerad. I'm Rachel, a friend of Dylan."

"It's good to meet you too, Rachel. Is Dylan OK? He didn't come for his appointment yesterday. I've been worried."

Rachel glanced at the open door. "Is there somewhere we can talk in private?" I led her downstairs to my room and closed the door behind us. "Dylan's in hospital. He tried to take his life yesterday."

"Oh my goodness, what happened? Have you spoken to him?"

"I've been with him since it happened. They're keeping him in for psychiatric evaluation. He asked me to come and see you. He speaks very highly of you."

"I'm very fond of him, Rachel."

"I can't think what made him do it. I mean, I know he's had some problems at work but other than that he's been visibly happy recently. We went climbing a couple of weeks ago and he said he had a completely new outlook on life. He said you had performed miracles with your needles. I asked him why he had done it but he didn't want to talk about it. He says you're the only person who will understand."

"Are you able to tell me what happened?"

"It was Sunday morning, really early. He left his flat and walked along the embankment to the bridge. He must have been really distressed. There were two girls there walking home from a party. They told the police that he had been standing in the middle of the bridge acting really weird and then all of a sudden he climbed over the railing…" She stopped for a moment, overcome with emotion. "They tried to stop him but he jumped before they could reach him. He was down in the water, being carried away by the current. He would have died, I'm sure of it, but there was a police boat and they fished him out. God knows what it was doing there at two o'clock in the morning, but they must have heard the screams from the bridge or maybe someone made a call, I don't know. If it wasn't for them… I don't even want to think about it. He wouldn't have lasted long in that water." Rachel wiped away her tears and shook her head in disbelief. "It upsets me so much to think how tormented he must have felt. I wish I could have been there to talk to him, to remind him how special he is."

* * *

A few weeks after Rachel's visit, Dylan came to see me. He seemed embarrassed and he was clearly agitated. He followed me down the stairs in silence and then perched awkwardly on the edge of the chair, his legs shaking. "I'm so sorry… I was doing really well and then I lost it… big time. I had the Christmas holidays to look forward to but instead of feeling good, I just felt desperately lonely and I was terrified that all that stuff I told you about was going to come out and I was worried about losing my job and I felt so ashamed of myself for making such a mess of everything and then..." He stopped suddenly, seemingly mesmerised by the rhythmic sound of his shoes drumming on the carpet.

"Keep going, Dylan, I'm listening."

"I got an email... It was Bronny, my cousin Rhys's mum. She said she was coming to London... that she wanted to see me. I panicked... I mean, I haven't seen her since it happened... Twenty years... I didn't know what to do. I just felt really, really scared... I couldn't get it out of my head. I got the Ritalin out and started necking it – I just had this overwhelming desire to escape from it all..." Dylan's hands were gripping the seat cushion and he was shaking.

"It's OK, I understand."

"I stayed up all night on Friday doing Ritalin – same thing on Saturday. By Sunday morning I was in a mess, I hadn't slept... All I could think about was putting an end to it... I couldn't face it... I went to the bridge and walked up and down... I felt confused... I thought I was going to pass out but then all of a sudden I just knew that I had to do it. I climbed over the barrier and... There were some people running towards me, shouting, but I wasn't afraid... I felt completely in control. I looked down at the water... and then I let myself go..." As he recalled the moment that he fell from the bridge, a stillness came over him, but almost immediately the look of terror returned. "The next thing I knew I was in the water and it was completely black. I didn't feel any pain or panic or anything, I didn't even feel the cold at first... It felt peaceful... and then suddenly I was totally overcome with panic. I knew I didn't want to die… I made it to the surface but I was getting carried away by the current. There were voices and a light and then I was being pulled towards a boat and someone was speaking to me and I was throwing up. I don't remember much else, it's all a bit of a blur…" Dylan ran his fingers through his hair and held the back of his head. "I nearly killed myself. It's not normal, is it?"

"We all do whatever we need to do at any given moment. There's no judgement. That's what happened. I'm glad you're still here."

* * *

In my earlier incarnation as a psychotherapist, my approach to helping Dylan would have been very different. I would have trawled through his past, picking apart patterns of thought and memory to understand the emotional and psychological cause of his distress. Since becoming a Five-Element acupuncturist, however, the way in which I work has changed. The only thing I know to be true, and therefore everything that I need to make a diagnosis, is what I see, hear, smell and feel in the treatment room. Everything else comes from the mind and is therefore questionable. When I started out as an acupuncturist, it was easy to become overly confident about my diagnostic skills. For example, I would meet a patient who smelled 'rotten', the odour associated with the Metal element, and then convince myself that I could perceive the other three sensory signals (the colour white, a weeping sound in the voice and a feeling of grief). I would then start asking leading questions in an attempt to make them collude with a diagnosis that I had reached using just one of the four legs of the stool. It's what we call 'leading the witness'. Worse still, I would think the signals were coming and going. I soon realised that it was *me* that was coming and going, not the ever-present sensory phenomena in front of me. As a therapist, where you choose to focus your attention is fundamentally important. As Fritz Perls, the founder of Gestalt therapy, which was the basis of my original training, wrote: "Lose your mind and come back to your senses." In Dylan's case, his putrid odour had immediately directed me to the Water element, but I knew that until I had done my due diligence, I wouldn't know for certain whether or not it was really the Causative Factor. To ascertain that, I had to check out the health of *all* five elements. Sometimes, they need a little encouragement to tell me how they're doing. For example, if I want to communicate with the Wood element, I have to speak its language, which is punchy and precise. When I interacted with Dylan in this way, there was no sense that he wanted to engage in a lively back-and-forth. He just froze. Equally, when I spoke to him in a sing-song voice, which is the sound produced by the Earth element, he just looked puzzled and I lost rapport. It was only when I remained still and spoke in a very measured, reassuring way that I could re-establish the relationship. The whole point of this investigative interaction is to establish what it is that the officials need. It's a forensic process that requires my full attention. As I probe, the patient responds from each of the five elements in the form of sensory signals, so it's essential for me to step back from the thinking mind and focus on what is actually happening in the room. If I am distracted by the siren call of the patient's story, those all-important signals will likely pass me by.

* * *

Dylan's experience of life was weighed down by a nagging sense of dread which, when it tipped the scales, compelled him either to retreat to a place of safety or release his pent-up tension in ways that were all too often unhealthy and self-destructive. When the Water element is out of balance – much like a dam that's either empty or unable to release its load – it no longer provides the reserves of power and flow for all the other officials to do their work. Our very existence is threatened and an alarm bell is activated, which we experience in the form of fear. The mind, also starved of the energy it needs, fails to understand that the fear comes from within and so looks to the outside world for its cause. The result is that everyday occurrences are seen as threatening. The mind is temporarily assuaged, because these events erroneously justify the feeling of panic, but ultimately it only serves to create more drama and further drains the well. For Dylan, the simple task of nipping out to buy some milk would have felt like a matter of life or death. Hanging off a sheer rock face without ropes, on the other hand, felt entirely natural, comforting even, because the inappropriate level of adrenaline that coursed through his veins felt right in that perilous pastime. In the same way, damaging cars gave him a sense of potency over his underlying terror and turbulent emotions, but it was a superficial balm for a much deeper wound. It wasn't until he tried to assert the ultimate control by taking his own life that he was finally able to see his actions for what they were. He had sought his own demise only to discover his appetite for life. He could finally see that the behaviour he had considered normal since childhood was actually driven by an unconscious fear of annihilation. It would be tempting to attribute Dylan's problems to events from his childhood, but although he had his challenges, they were certainly not out of the ordinary. Events can trigger and exacerbate our struggles; however in order to heal ourselves we need to look beyond our stories and become aware of how we function, both in and out of balance. Dylan's imbalance in the Water element put every part of his body, mind and spirit into survival mode and this fundamentally affected how he experienced his life. Fear itself is not a problem – it's what enables us to cross the road without getting hit by a car, after all – but once it is taken to extremes, it becomes a cause of disease.

* * *

In the weeks following his attempted suicide, I felt the need to keep a watchful eye on Dylan. I gave him whatever I could in the way of advice and reassurance, but I was fully aware that there was a limit to what I could do for him with words alone. The qualities that he most needed to set him on the path to recovery would come from within, so the effect of verbal counselling would likely only be superficial and fleeting. It is the Bladder and Kidney officials, when they are working well, that provide us with an innate and enduring sense of safety and power. In light of this, I decided to up the treatments on the Water element to twice a week, in order to give all his officials the extra support they needed. Within a few weeks, Dylan began to demonstrate a level of resilience and personal awareness that I had not seen in him before. Little had changed in the circumstances of his day-to-day existence but, after years of inner turmoil, he was finally able to live his life by design rather than compulsion. I told him that if he ever felt in danger of losing control again, he should contact me immediately. He seemed surprised but grateful for the offer. Apparently, even a modest gesture of warmth and kindness helped this fearful man to tap into his own latent capacity to feel safe and secure within himself. To this day, Dylan still comes for treatment in the knowledge that, despite his brush with death and the seismic shift that it provoked in him, his fight or flight response is still easily triggered. However, coming back into balance has given him a new perspective that has enabled him to tame his more destructive impulses and channel his considerable reserves of energy into more constructive pursuits.

'Illuminated Sea' is an acupuncture point located on the Kidney meridian, just under the inner ankle bone. The Chinese character evokes the image of a large body of water lit by the light of the moon. It represents the profound sense of peace that we experience when we truly understand the depth of our being. Dylan's transition from a state of extreme trauma to one of relative tranquillity was nothing short of extraordinary. Maintaining balance in mind, body and spirit requires him to be constantly vigilant. He still has the occasional drama, but he has made a remarkable leap forward from where he started not so long ago. In the space between fear and fearlessness, he has found stillness and strength.

3

LOATHSOME JAW

*

I rarely have time between appointments to gather my thoughts, but on this particular morning, there had been a cancellation, so I was busy catching up on emails when the buzzer rang to announce the arrival of my next patient. I looked at my watch. It was eleven forty-five. I opened my diary to see who was coming at twelve. Tarik. I smiled and returned my attention to my inbox. Shortly afterwards, the buzzer sounded again and then barely a minute later, there was a knock on the door. It was Eszter.

"Sorry, Gerad, but Tarik is upstairs and he's driving me nuts. He pushed his way through the front door as I was showing someone out and now he's pacing around the reception area like a tiger, asking when you'll be ready for him."

"Eszter, please! It's only eleven fifty! You know Tarik always comes early. Ask him to take a seat in the waiting room. I'll be up shortly."

"I already tried that but he's not having it. He keeps asking me to check whether or not you know that he's here." I stopped what I was doing and walked upstairs, followed closely by a slightly breathless Eszter, who was clearly excited by the possibility of some drama to spice up her morning. Sure enough, there was Tarik who, despite his diminutive stature, was standing imperiously in the middle of the reception area with a tangible air of impatience.

"Ah, Gerard! Let's get started, shall we? I have a lunch meeting right after this and I cannot be late." I forced a grin to conceal my irritation. Even after decades in this job, it never ceases to amaze me how certain patients can instantly trigger a reaction in me that confirms my diagnosis. With Tarik, it was always anger and annoyance that I felt, which was perfectly in line with the emotion associated with the Wood element. Nevertheless, I resisted taking the bait and steeled myself for the session.

"Good morning, Tarik. I'm delighted to see you as always but you do realise you're early, don't you?"

"My appointment is at ten," he replied, tapping his watch. I made a point of turning to look at the clock on the wall and then smiled at Tarik without saying anything.

"I just wanted you to know that I'm here, Gerard. I'm never sure whether she actually tells you or not." He glanced condescendingly at Eszter, who was quietly seething behind the reception desk. "She told me she buzzed you, but judging by previous experiences, I'm guessing the buzzer doesn't work."

"It's working just fine, Tarik. Anyway, since I'm here now, we may as well get started." Before I could gesture for him to follow me, Tarik had disappeared into the hallway and down the stairs. I took a deep breath, winked at Eszter and followed in his wake. Although Tarik was only about five foot five, there was a power and presence about him that you couldn't ignore. Watching him walk down the stairs with such confidence, push open the door to my treatment room and take control of the space was a sight to behold. I imagined this feisty Napoleonic figure out in the world, sweeping everyone and everything aside in that same self-assured manner. I'm sure many people would have interpreted his behaviour as aggressive or arrogant, but as I had come to realise over the years, there was no malign intent. It was just his way.

The season of the Wood element is spring and its remit is to kickstart each new cycle of life. After the long winter months, spring bursts into life and activates Nature's plan with absolute clarity and confidence. There is no hesitancy or indecision. It is a full and free expression of life: vital, impatient and unwavering. But it is also flexible. Just as water finds the path of least resistance, so too the shoots that emerge from the once-dormant seeds find their way around seemingly insurmountable obstacles with consummate ease and knowing. When the officials of the Wood element are functioning as they should, this blend of outward force and yielding grace is mirrored within us. When they are not, one or other of these qualities becomes exaggerated, resulting in inappropriate levels of timidity or assertiveness. The former feels like resignation. The latter, which could often be seen in Tarik's demeanour, feels like anger. In fact, it is simply an expression of frustration, born of plans that are clearly seen but never realised.

Tarik strode into the room, hung his jacket on the coat rack, folded his scarf in three and placed it on the floor beside the armchair, just as he always did. For Tarik, routine and precision were everything. Having completed his ritual, he then settled into the chair and looked me squarely in the eyes. I returned the look. Neither of us flinched.

"So, how have you been, Tarik?"

"The headaches are back in full force. Not good."

"I'm sorry to hear that. Has anything in your life changed recently?"

"Spare me the psychotherapy, please. Just fix me. And remember that I need to leave bang on time today." Tarik had come to me several years before complaining of fatigue, migraines and low mood. Typically, I ask a new patient to come once a week for the first month so I can get on top of the symptoms, but Tarik wanted to do things his way. "Coming weekly doesn't work for me," he had told me. "I'll come once a month."

The patient/practitioner relationship has an interesting dynamic. According to the classical texts, the acupuncturist must not mother or nurse the patient. Rather, the task is to find the fastest way to diagnose and treat in accordance with natural law. However, the ancient teachings also stress the importance of creating an environment in which love and compassion are present. It is said that when two people come together in the name of change, the five spirits descend and healing occurs. The acupuncture needle is the conduit for that change. I realised right away that Tarik's tendency to challenge me would make it difficult to maintain rapport, so I decided to meet him in the middle and cede a little ground without losing my authority. Right from the start, he wanted to know exactly what I was doing and why. It wasn't so much curiosity as a need to understand how I planned to help him. I'm always happy to share my knowledge, but there's only so much detail I can provide while focusing on the task at hand. So, one day, in the midst of his questioning, I suggested that he watch some of the training films on my acupuncture school's website. It was a throwaway comment but Tarik took it as a challenge. Within months, he had garnered a detailed understanding of Five-Element theory and proudly told me that he could now diagnose family and friends with ease.

"My wife smells of overripe fruit," he announced one day. "Earth! Simple. I should be doing your job." On the whole, his new-found knowledge was playful but, in his determination to learn as much as he possibly could, he ended up drawing on conflicting strands of information from distinctly different schools of acupuncture. The result was a hybrid theory that only made sense when it happened to collide with the truth. I was tempted to correct him but I knew that it would serve no purpose. What interested me was not so much the content of his theory, as flawed as it was, but the fact that he was so wedded to it. He read everything he could find until he had developed a theoretical framework that made sense to him, and then he wouldn't budge from it.

"OK, Tarik, let's see what's going on with you. Shoes

and socks off, please. Trousers too, unless you can roll them up above your knees." I gestured towards the treatment couch, but he pushed himself back into the chair and crossed his legs.

"As you know very well by now, my trousers are tailor made. Rolling them up is out of the question. Now, Gerard! Before I get on the couch, tell me how *you* are." Tarik always got my name wrong and he knew it, but for him there was only one correct spelling of the name and that was that. Who was I to argue?

"I'm well, thank you, Tarik. It's been a busy time."

"Yes, I noticed. I've been following you on social media. Travelling, throwing dinner parties, walking your dogs... Where on earth does work fit into all of that?" He grinned at me. "Anyway, I've been thinking, Gerard. You don't charge enough. I've been coming to see you for years and your fee hasn't gone up in all that time." In fact, I had increased my fee some time before but had chosen not to tell him to avoid any potential backlash. In retrospect, it was a mistake. By allowing myself to be intimidated by him, I had fuelled the very thing that he needed to address.

"Thank you, Tarik. How much do you think I should charge?"

"I think the right price is a hundred and fifty." He paused for a moment as he untied his laces and removed his shoes and socks. "No more than that, or people will think you're being greedy." He rose to his feet, unbuckled his belt and painstakingly removed his trousers to reveal a pair of sun-starved legs. "But definitely no less because let's face it, you're not getting any younger, are you?" This was one of many moments when I felt Tarik's generosity, though it was often couched in bossiness. Despite his bullish manner, which all too often caused offence, he only ever wanted the best for people. I left the room briefly to wash my hands and when I came back Tarik was standing next to the treatment couch with his hands on his hips.

"When are you going to get a stool, Gerard? This thing is ridiculously high."

* * *

Tarik had left his native Bosnia in 1996, not long after the end of the war that had torn his country apart. He had spent fifteen years in Copenhagen before moving to London in the late nineties with his wife Tilde and their two daughters. Tilde had been born and brought up in Denmark but she had long harboured ambitions to live in London, so when she was offered a job with a firm of British architects, she jumped at the opportunity. They settled in quickly and Tarik took great pleasure in adopting the English way of life, albeit a somewhat idealised version of it. He loved the royal family and developed an obsession for the aristocracy, whose style and speech he tried to mimic, with mixed results. He began dressing in blazers and brogues and, despite the inevitable remnants of an accent that betrayed his origins, his manner of speaking gradually morphed into something resembling that of a wartime radio announcer. No doubt there were those that sneered at his attempts to integrate so fully with his adopted country, but I found it endearing. And courageous. To reinvent yourself is never easy, particularly when the need to do so has been forced on you by the most appalling of circumstances.

In the years before his move, Tarik had worked for an art dealer in Copenhagen who had taken him under his wing and taught him the tricks of the trade. Soon after arriving in London, he decided to follow in the footsteps of his mentor and began working in the art scene. He networked tirelessly and prided himself on being connected to all the right people. Within a few years, he was making good money but, despite his achievements, he couldn't let go of the nagging discontent of being on the 'wrong side' of the business. Instead of producing the art, which had been his dream since childhood, he was peddling it, and even though he was respected by his peers, he was incapable of seeing himself as a success. The intense frustration that he experienced, the outcome of the feeling that he simply couldn't move forward with his life in the way that he wanted to, was something that troubled him immensely and seemed to trap him in an endless cycle of unfulfilled dreams.

"Tagore expressed it perfectly," he told me once in a rare moment of philosophical reflection. "'I have spent my days stringing and unstringing my instrument but the song that I came to sing remains unsung.'" Tarik's voice was revealing. Even when he was quoting poetry, it sounded like he was telling me off. Short, clipped sentences thrown at me one after another like a volley of tennis balls. This is the sound of the Wood element struggling to grow with ease, and it can often feel a little combative. Nevertheless, if I want to maintain rapport with a patient whose Causative Factor is in the Wood element, it's essential for me to respond in kind. No jokes, no sympathy. Just questions and answers, clear and exact.

"What is it about being an artist that appeals to you, Tarik?"

"I'm good at it, Gerard. I painted portraits when I was a kid. People said I was a natural."

"Are you still making portraits?"

"Of course not, I'm far too busy. Anyway, it's impossible."

"Impossible?"

"I need a studio."

"There are plenty of studios in London."

"I need something with space and light. And it needs to be in a good location."

"Something like this?"

"With respect, Gerard, I couldn't spend all day in here."

"It seems such a waste, Tarik. You say that you love art but you're not producing anything. Not even sketches?"

"I don't do sketches, Gerard. I'm a painter."

"I'm a fan of the bite-sized-chunks approach to life. Wouldn't it be interesting to try to start again, even in a small way, and see if it takes off?"

"What's the point? I haven't been to art school. I don't have any training."

"But you told me that you have a natural talent."

"I do, but there are thousands of artists out there. I can't possibly compete with them." Tarik shut down everything I suggested. It was as if he had already accepted that he would never realise his dream, so why even try?

"Tarik, if creative success is so important to you, why not set yourself a goal and take the necessary steps to get there?"

"Steps?"

"Yes. One step at a time. Here's a suggestion. I have a patient who used to be a lawyer but is now working as an artist. She has a large studio in North London. Would you like me to ask if she'd be willing to meet with you and tell you how she made the transition? It might give you the inspiration you need." Tarik shuffled uncomfortably in his chair. As he did so, I became aware once again of that familiar rancid odour, the smell of soured milk, which is the alarm bell of the Wood element in distress.

"I'll think about it."

* * *

I vividly remember the first time I met Tarik. It was at my old clinic in New Bond Street, where a large sweeping staircase led from the reception area to a galleried mezzanine with half a dozen treatment rooms. As I walked down the staircase that day, I was met by a fierce-looking figure with a furrowed brow and tightly clenched fists. He was immaculately dressed in a green tweed suit and a check shirt with matching blue tie and pocket square.

"Gerard!" he barked.

"Yes, that's me. You must be Tarik." I held out my hand, expecting a bold and confident grip but was met instead with a softness and warmth that communicated something very different. I led him up to the treatment room, whereupon he told me what I would be doing for him and how it was going to work. I found it fascinating how clearly he envisioned the outcome of something he knew nothing about. Right from the start, his demeanour was forthright and fearless, but I had the sense that this seemingly natural and abundant self-confidence was rooted in timidity.

In the years that followed, I would come to know a man who was deeply loyal, both to me personally and to the treatment process. Had anyone said something negative about me or my work, I have no doubt that he would have defended me to the hilt. But this fierce sense of loyalty would often tip into intransigence. Everything had to be done in the right way, and the 'right way' was always *his* way. Other people were entitled to have their own opinions, but they were wrong. I remember him describing how he micromanaged his decorator. He would follow him up the ladder to ensure that he cut in correctly with the line of paint between the wall and ceiling. The poor man put up with this for weeks until he finally dared to offer an opinion, at which point he was summarily dismissed. There was something rather intriguing about this attention to detail. It was deeply annoying when you were the one being scrutinised, yet it wasn't meant as criticism. Indeed, there was a goodness and greatness about Tarik, but being tied to the mast of righteousness meant that he struggled to be at peace with himself and the world around him.

A few years after he first started coming to see me for treatment, Tarik invited me for lunch. I am very careful to maintain appropriate boundaries with my patients, so I thanked him for the invitation but declined, citing practitioner/patient norms.

"Gerard! You're talking nonsense. You're coming for lunch and that's final." Once again, I allowed his assertive manner to get the better of my judgement and agreed to schedule it for the following week. It was a fascinating experience to see him in the real world, acting just as I imagined he would. Despite his height, Tarik walked with such pace and purpose that people swerved to get out of his way. It was like the apocryphal parting of the waters. We made our way to a bustling Chinese restaurant not far from the clinic, which Tarik told me was the best in town. On arrival, he strode in and stood with his chest puffed out as if he owned the place. A rather fragile-looking man appeared and asked if we had a reservation.

"We do."

"Your name?"

"Dragovic."

"I'm sorry?"

"Dragovic!"

The man checked his watch and started leafing through a large diary covered in handwritten names. "Could you spell that for me, please?"

"Oh, for goodness sake!" Tarik snatched the book and ran his finger down the page. "There! Dragovic. Two people." The man was clearly intimidated but he calmly invited us to follow him to our table, which was in the middle of the room. Tarik took one look at it and shook his head. "No, this won't do. I specifically asked for a table by the window." He scanned the room like a bird of prey until his eyes settled on a large table in the far corner by a large floor-to-ceiling window. "We'll take that table over there."

"I'm very sorry, sir, but that's for a party of four. And it's reserved." Tarik folded his arms and stared at him with undisguised irritation.

"Well, I suggest you unreserve it, then." The man opened his mouth to speak but thought better of it. And, just like that, the table that Tarik wanted was ours. As comical as this scenario might sound, I felt deeply uneasy. I was already struggling to cross the personal/professional boundary and the manner in which he had treated this man only served to exacerbate my discomfort. Nevertheless, my role as a practitioner of this system of medicine is to observe what is inappropriate about someone, not to judge their behaviour. Tarik was either oblivious to the way he made others feel or he was just plain rude. Whichever it was, I banked the information, settled into my chair and waited for Tarik to tell me what I was going to eat.

* * *

The lunch at the Chinese restaurant, although uncomfortable, had been instructive from a clinical point of view because it confirmed certain behaviours that I had observed in the privacy of the treatment room, most notably his quick temper. Tarik wasn't someone who harboured ill will towards others but, in his skewed perception of the world, he saw everyone and everything as an obstacle standing in his way. This point of view had no basis in reality but, fuelled as it was by a powerful imbalance inside, it would have seemed very real to him. The frustration that he felt fomented a simmering rage that frequently rose to the surface in inappropriate outbursts. Although the release of anger would give him a fleeting sense of relief, it actually backfired because it legitimised his feelings of injustice and despair. Our lunch together would have been meticulously planned and he would have expected everything to unfold exactly as he had envisaged it. The same was true of his visits to my clinic. If anything delayed him, such as a traffic jam or a sudden downpour, it would awaken his demons. Rather than adapt to the situation, he would boil with rage and take it out on anyone who was unfortunate enough to be around him. By the time he reached the clinic, he would be as black as thunder and inevitably it was poor Eszter who took the hit. However charming she tried to be (and charm was not her strong point), Tarik could only see her as an irritation, an unnecessary and inefficient intermediary between him and me.

"You should get rid of that awful woman," he told me. "She has no idea what she's doing. And she *still* gets my name wrong even though I've been coming here for years. It's infuriating."

"I'm sure she's trying her best."

"Well, her best isn't good enough."

Most of us rarely question the origin of our emotions. Whether we are happy or sad, we assume it is because someone or something has made us feel that way. In fact, our emotional state is a mirror of the health and balance of the five elements within us. In other words, the way we react to situations says more about us than the apparent cause of our reaction. Anger, the emotion that relates to the Wood element, is a perfectly healthy and useful tool when it is employed appropriately. When they are functioning well, the Wood officials enable us to grow with the same kind of effortless grace as new shoots in the springtime. When they lose their natural equilibrium, however, we are no longer able to see a way forward and this natural ease and flexibility gives way to an angry, unbending force fuelled by frustration. We advance through coercion or, if our overbearing manner fails to yield the desired results, give up completely and sink into a state of apathy and resignation. The life that Tarik longed for was etched indelibly in his mind, but he simply didn't know how to take the first step towards its realisation. Every failed attempt was yet more evidence of a dark and obstructive world in which only others thrived. Frustration and adversity became his norm, and a sense of hopelessness shrouded any trace of optimism for the life that, deep down, he knew could be his.

* * *

My relationship with Tarik was very clear. I was there to

serve him and he paid me for this service. That may sound obvious, but many of my patients want far more than a transactional relationship. A counsellor, a crutch, or simply someone to whom they can talk about their struggles. In Tarik's case, the contract was established right from the start. He had been referred to me by his doctor who, he hastened to add, was one of the finest in London, and he was here to be fixed. Period.

"I only go to the best, Gerard," he told me and then held my gaze, waiting for some recognition of the compliment.

"I'm honoured, Tarik, thank you." Our relationship continued in this way for years. Occasionally I would attempt to go a little bit deeper, not only because I wanted to eradicate the symptoms that still persisted, but also because I sensed that there was something else waiting to come to the surface. In one of our very first sessions, he had told me that he lost some family members in the Bosnian war, but that was all the information I had and Tarik had made it very clear that it was not something he wanted to talk about. "That's all in the past, Gerard. Let's leave it there, OK?" So although my wish was to help him in any way that I could, I backed off, afraid of the reaction that it might provoke. In retrospect, it was a failure on my part.

Early in 2016, Tarik sent me an email to ask if he could postpone his appointment. In all the years that I had known him, he had never changed or missed a session, so I was concerned. I offered him an alternative date and asked if everything was OK. The response was abrupt.

"I'm fine. See you next week." The following Wednesday, Tarik walked into my room and sat down in the chair without taking his jacket or scarf off.

"I have bad news, Gerard. Tilde has cancer."

"Oh, Tarik, I'm so sorry."

"It started in the breast but it's spread. She has secondaries in her liver and bones. They say there's nothing they can do about it." I was completely thrown by what he had told me. Lost for words, I reached over and rested my hand on his. He stared at the floor and brushed my hand away as his eyes welled up with tears. "I failed my family and now I've failed Tilde and the girls." This sudden moment of introspection, as shocking as it was, was the first time Tarik had revealed so much as a hint of weakness. It was also an opportunity. I had avoided some of the more difficult conversations with him in the past, preferring collusion to confrontation, but this was not a time for me and my personal experience of him to get in the way.

"Do you want to say more about that, Tarik? What do you mean by 'failing'?" He looked up at me, tears streaming down his face, and began to sob uncontrollably.

* * *

A few days later, I received an email from Tarik saying that he would like to start coming once a week. I agreed without hesitation and assured him that I would do whatever I could to help him. When he arrived the following week, he told me in detail about his new self-development programme and support network, of which I was to be a part.

"To help my family, I need to be at my absolute best. Failure is not an option." It seemed that the man who believed he had failed his family was now going into overdrive to make up for his imagined shortcomings. "First off, my meditation teacher thinks I have an energy block. Let's start with that."

"Tarik, sometimes blocks are there because of things from our past that we haven't dealt with. The needles work wonders but sharing our more challenging experiences can really help. I'm sure we can agree that our work together has been helpful but maybe this is the time to take it to the next level?" This was a risk. I was speaking directly to Tarik, not his fiercely defended construct, and I was unsure how it would land. "Last week you talked about failing your family. What did you mean by that?" He was silent for a few moments but when he looked up I noticed something that I had not seen before. Behind those glowering eyes was a deeply wounded, vulnerable man.

"Imagine what it's like not to be able to protect the people you love, Gerard. To be completely powerless to do anything. I was in Sarajevo working for my uncle when the war broke out. I should have got out of there right away – but it all happened so quickly. Before we could organise ourselves, the city was under siege. We were fired at day and night by snipers. I was terrified. We all were. But all I could think about was my family. About a year and a half into the siege, my uncle paid the soldiers so I could get out through the secret tunnel that had just been finished.

I walked for days under the cover of darkness and then one day I ran into the Serbs. They knew right away that I was a Bosniak. They threw me in one of the camps. There were several thousand of us there. We were beaten. Badly beaten. Terrible things happened. Unimaginable things. There was nothing I could do. Nothing. I should have been at home, protecting them. My mother. My sisters. And then one day it was over." He stopped for a moment and stared at the floor.

"Your family?"

"They killed them. All of them. My mother and father were shot. My sisters were beaten and raped. Then they were killed. I wasn't there to protect them." He lifted his head and looked me directly in the eyes. "I vowed never to let anyone take my freedom away again. And I vowed that I would never again fail my family." I was completely at a loss for what to say. This was not the first time that a patient of mine had told me about a tragedy in their life, but never before had I heard such horrifying recollections told with such force and fury. As I watched this brave man facing up to the memory of such unthinkable grief and suffering, I felt a profound connection with him. For the first time since we had met, I sensed that I was seeing the real Tarik and I knew in that moment what it was that he needed. It was a turning point for us both.

* * *

Tilde's health continued to deteriorate but Tarik was undeterred. He researched every available treatment, conventional and experimental, and consulted with every specialist he could get hold of, wherever they happened to be. Armed with this information, he then mapped out a strategy for Tilde's recovery in minute detail. Dates, locations, specialists, medication, surgery, convalescence – all of it was laid out in meticulous detail on a spreadsheet that he presented to me.

"I'm taking Tilde to Boston next week to see a consultant who is working on a cutting-edge treatment. The girls are coming, too. We may be there for a while, so I've arranged for a private tutor." Tarik's indomitable spirit was back in full force, fuelled by his determination to save Tilde. He fought for her survival like a warrior and if anyone said anything that he perceived as defeatist or unhelpful, they were out. His way was the right way, the outcome was certain, and nobody could tell him anything different.

'Loathsome Jaw' is an acupuncture point found on the Gallbladder meridian and is located on the side of the head. It's where the muscles of the temple ripple and tense when we commit to something with absolute determination. Tarik had felt stuck, unable to realise his most cherished dream of becoming an artist, but the prospect of losing his wife to cancer suddenly freed him from the inertia and indecision that had plagued his life. Sadly, it had taken a life-and-death situation to set him on a new course.

* * *

Almost a year after he had left for Boston, Tarik called

with the news of Tilde's death. He said that he would be returning to London the following month and asked if he could come to see me after the dust had settled. He sounded devastated but, curiously, the predominant impression I got was not one of resignation, as I had expected, but liberation. In fact, it was another six months before he got in touch. On the day that he was due to come in for treatment, I had nipped out to buy a sandwich when I suddenly caught sight of him, weaving his way in and out of the people in his path with an ease that I hadn't seen in him before. As he approached, he shot me a look, did a double take and then stopped.

"Gerard? Yes, it's you! Why aren't you working?" I held up my sandwich.

"Great to see you, Tarik. Where are you off to? You look like you're on a mission."

"I'm off to Mayfair to pick up a suit. Can't stop. I'll see you at three. Don't be late!" Before I had time to reply he was off, tearing down the street towards Piccadilly for a rendez-vous with his favourite tailor. I walked back to the clinic, polished off my sandwich and welcomed my next patient, a woman in her twenties who was coming to me for the first time. At two forty-five the buzzer went off as I was needling a point on her abdomen.

"Oh, is our time up?" she asked anxiously.

"Not at all, it's just my next patient. He's early." Five minutes later, the buzzer went off again and at two fifty-five, just as my patient was putting her coat on to leave, there was a knock at the door. I opened it, expecting to see Eszter, only to find Tarik brandishing a suit carrier emblazoned with the words 'Anderson and Sheppard'.

"Best tailors in town, Gerard. Prince Charles gets his suits made there, did you know that?"

"I didn't, no. Did Eszter not ask you to wait upstairs for me?"

"She did but I was excited to see you." I stepped aside to allow my patient to leave, ushered Tarik in and walked over to the filing cabinet to retrieve my notes from our last session together. When I turned around, he was sitting on the arm of the chair, his scarf thrown over his shoulder. I sat down and gestured for Tarik to do the same. He dropped the scarf onto the floor beside him, sunk into the armchair and crossed his legs.

"I'm so sorry for your loss, Tarik."

"Thank you, Gerard. It's been a very difficult time but life must go on. My focus now is the girls. It's been really tough for them, so I decided to give us all a fresh start. I've made an offer on a little house next to a river, just south of Oxford. I'm going to work remotely from now on and I've managed to get the girls into the best school in the area. I think it'll do us all a power of good to be out of the city, away from all the memories." Tarik's voice had changed. The staccato timbre that had always made me feel like he was ticking me off had given way to a softer, warmer tone. He told me about the final weeks with Tilde and how, when she died, he had experienced a profound sense of peace before the grief took hold.

"I did everything I could, Gerard, and I'm proud of that, but it's over now. It's time to look forward and I'm determined to provide the girls with all the love and security that they deserve." I was struck by the calm aura that surrounded this normally agitated man. He had accepted his new reality without a hint of self-pity or anger. The instinct of the warrior was still there, but it seemed to have been tempered by a willingness to adapt to changing circumstances. It reminded me of a point on the Liver meridian that perfectly exemplifies the flexibility of Wood when it is in balance. 'Great Esteem', also known as 'Great Meekness', not only gives us the strength to move forward in life with resoluteness and vigour, but also the wisdom and humility to surrender when necessary. Tarik's younger years had been exceptionally difficult, but rather than allow the rest of his life to be defined by the trauma that he had suffered, he had created a prosperous life for himself through sheer force of will. I thought back to the day that we had met for lunch and finally understood the mindset of the man who had only ever seen life as a series of battles to be won. It was somewhat ironic that the greatest of them all, the battle to save his wife, was the very thing that would bring him peace. Here was a man, beset by so many challenges, flourishing in the aftermath of defeat. 'Gate of Hope' is the final point on the Liver meridian. The Chinese character for this point is a person lying on soft, dewy grass, bathed in the light of the moon filtering through the open weave of delicate muslin. This beautiful image illustrates our natural tendency to surrender to the unknown as we wait for the dawn and the promise of the day to come.

"I'm so pleased you're able to look forward, Tarik. I know how much loss you've experienced in your life. It takes a lot of courage to keep going."

He sat upright and slapped his thighs with the palms of his hands.

"It will never be the same without Tilde, but the best way I can honour her memory is to give the girls the life we had planned for them. That's all that matters now." The change in our interaction was remarkable. It was as if he had freed himself from his myopic perspective and embraced the limitless possibilities of life.

"What's the house like, Tarik? It sounds rather magical."

"It's everything I could wish for. Oh, and by the way, there's an outhouse that I'm going to convert into a studio. You can be my first sitter if you like."

* * *

Tarik's transformation had a profound impact on me because it was a textbook illustration of the way in which someone can find the natural point of balance between two opposing states: the searing pain of loss, with its inexorable pull to the past, and the joyous feeling of a rebirth, replete with purpose and possibility. The natural cycle of destruction and creation had played out in front of my eyes. For many years, Tarik continued to see me at the change of each season. One day, just as autumn was giving way to the first days of winter, he turned up for his appointment looking pale and drawn.

"Just so you know, Gerard, I'm not paying you for this session."

"Why's that, Tarik?"

"Well, I've been doing some research and it appears that in ancient China, people only paid the acupuncturist if there was nothing wrong with them. The acupuncturist was responsible for keeping the community in good health through preventative treatment, so if someone was sick, they wouldn't have to pay."

"Fair enough, Tarik. You probably also read that everyone paid an annual retainer, so how about we settle on a figure and take it from there?"

"You have an answer for everything, don't you?" Tarik's inimitable spirit remained unchanged, but what once would have come across as belligerence had evolved into a playful sparring that was fun to engage with. As his mental and physical health continued to improve, I noticed that he only made important decisions for himself and his daughters when he felt well in himself. There seemed to be a recognition that the place of balance he had come to know was the launchpad for healthy choices, and the outcome of these choices showed him that his life was unfolding in the manner of his choosing: just and exact.

4

WELCOME FRAGRANCE

*

Martha was a theatre agent and she cut a suitably impressive figure. She was in her early sixties, but a healthy diet, vigorous exercise and an appetite for younger men had all combined to give her the aura and physique of a forty-year-old. Her skin had a youthful lustre, and apart from a handful of grey hairs, her thick, shoulder-length mane had maintained its original auburn glow. Her outfits were elegant and stylish, but on closer inspection there was always something out of place. Creases that spoke of a certain neglect, a hole in a jumper, a hastily chosen scarf that didn't match the rest of her outfit. The most jarring thing about her, however, was her apparent disconnection from everyone and everything around her. She would stare ahead as if in a trance, apparently unaware of whatever was unfolding in real time. Gestures would go unnoticed and words seemed to pass her by, before eventually eliciting a long-awaited response. It was like talking to someone on the other side of the world with an agonisingly long time delay.

It was late October when she first came to see me and, as the last vestiges of autumn fell from the trees, there was a familiar feeling of melancholy in the air. Martha had been referred to me by a friend who worked in theatre. She seemed troubled, he told me. Full of regrets and resentments. Mournful, even. Indeed, as I walked into the waiting room to collect her, I was struck by the unusually heavy atmosphere. She was sitting by the window at the far end of the room, pulling at her hair. She seemed completely unaware of my presence.

"Good morning, you must be Martha." She turned her head towards me and stared blankly. I stepped forward and tried to make eye contact. "Hello? Martha? I'm Gerad."

She cocked her head to one side and then broke into a smile as if she had suddenly recognised a long lost friend. "Hello. I hate this season. It's so depressing." I waited while she gathered her things and then led her down to my room. She sunk into the armchair, straightened her blouse and started brushing hairs from the sleeves of her jacket. Once she was satisfied that there were none left, she removed the jacket and then, to my surprise, let it drop to the floor beside her chair. I took my seat, placed the clipboard on my knees and clicked my pen to signal that the session had begun.

"I'm not exactly sure why I'm here," she announced. "I mean, I've had lots of therapy over the years and it's been pretty shit to be honest, besides which I'm not someone who needs a lot of attention but when things get really…"

"Martha, I'm sorry to interrupt you but I'd like to explain how I work before we get into the detail." Once again she stared at me with a completely blank expression. I wasn't sure if she was furious with me for interrupting, confused by what I was saying or just plain disinterested. "I'm aware that you were referred to me by my friend, Richard, but just so you know, anything you tell me in this room is confidential. Nothing you say about him or anyone else we both know will affect the way I think about them."

"What, like if I tell you that Richard's been a naughty boy at the theatre?" She took a swig from her water bottle, winked at me and snortled, which caused the water to stream out of her nose. She spluttered an apology and wiped the water from her face with her sleeve.

"What would you most like to get from having treatment, Martha?"

"Well, I was telling Richard about the shitty situation with my family and he suggested I come to you for some help in working it all out."

"Of course, no problem, but is there anything else you'd like me to help you with?" Another vacant stare put us both into a freeze frame. "Martha?" Her name seemed to hang in the air as she looked at me, apparently unaware that I was waiting for a response. She seemed lost, and it was a good ten seconds before she finally found her way back and met my gaze, as if for the first time.

"I don't really know what's on offer. I just don't want to feel so dark and hopeless about everything."

"Just for a moment, let's imagine that your family situation has been resolved. Is there anything you've always wanted to do but never quite achieved? Or maybe you have a habit that bugs you but you can't seem to shake it?" No sooner had the words left my mouth than I wondered why I had uttered them. Asking abstract questions wasn't going to help, it would likely only exacerbate this feeling of disconnection. So why was I doing this? My behaviour seemed to be telling me something about my new patient. Rather than sit back and experience the phenomena of the person in front of me, I was trying to force a connection through my questioning.

Being connected to ourselves, the people around us and the world at large is something that most of us take for granted, but there are times when all of our normal reference points are lost. All of a sudden we struggle to make sense of who we are, where we are and why we are here. We often experience this when grieving, as we adjust to the loss of a loved one, a possession or even a part of our identity. Over time, most of us come to terms with our new reality, but for some, this abstracted, empty state becomes the norm. It comes about because the inner component that connects us to the universal matrix is faulty. We feel alienated and confused as we desperately search for something to hold onto, something that will give us a sense of connection and belonging.

In ancient Chinese philosophy, the Metal element was considered to be the means by which we find our place in life and maintain a relationship with our maker. The concept of being connected to a deity is found in most religions, but in the Taoist tradition, the relationship is with the entirety of existence rather than a singular divine being. The Metal element, which is associated with the lungs and the large intestine, facilitates and supports this connection. In the West, we tend to focus on the physiological aspects of being alive. For the ancient Chinese, however, the body was simply the tangible realm of a multi-faceted existence, consisting of body, mind and spirit. Seen from the perspective of Western medicine, the lungs inhale oxygen and then exhale carbon dioxide. Seen through the lens of Chinese medicine, the inhalation of breath is the physical representation of "receiving the heavenly 'qi'", which is how the Lung official ensures that we are nourished on all three levels. In the same way, the expulsion of carbon dioxide in the out-breath is a physical representation of the excretion of waste under the remit of the Large Intestine official. What was going on with Martha? Was this trance-like state an inability to receive me and my questions or was she so constipated in body, mind and spirit that there was simply no room for anything new?

"OK, Martha, let's start with your work and your home life. Can you give me a sense of your day-to-day routine?"

She jutted her chin forward and moved her head from side to side as if she were trying to make room for my question. "It's shit. I'm living in a rented flat with one of my sons who's just broken up with his partner. Thank God. Horrible woman. Anyway, at the age of thirty-two, he's decided he needs to come home to Mummy. He's grossly overweight and if I'm honest, I struggle with that." She seemed disturbed by what she had just told me and looked away.

"What about your work?"

"I'm a theatre agent. Been doing it for over thirty years and I'm sick of it. It pays the bills and I'm grateful for that but I'm so tired of working with second-rate actors."

"Was this something you wanted to do or did you fall into it?"

"Are you kidding me? I worked my butt off to get into the business but had I known how dull and uninspiring it was going to be, I wouldn't have bothered." She scooped up her hair and started running it through her hands over and over again, releasing a flurry of dandruff that fell onto the shoulder pads of her jacket. Pretty much everything that came out of Martha's mouth was laced with negativity but the most jarring thing of all was the force with which she dismissed everything and everyone, including me. There was a tangible air of disappointment and disgust, and this, combined with the blank look, added an unsettling edge to our interaction.

"Is there anything that you enjoy in your life right now?"

"My AA meetings."

"Alcoholics Anonymous?"

"Yes, I love the feeling of belonging. They're all fucked up but there's no judgement and I feel valued. AA is my family." While she was talking about AA, Martha had visibly softened, but it was short-lived. No sooner had she relaxed than she uncrossed her legs and leaned forward in her chair to get my full attention. "Are we going to talk about why I'm here?"

"Yes, of course. Please tell me."

Martha exhaled between pursed lips and then filled

her lungs in preparation for what she was about to offload into the room. "So here's the thing. My mother is an absolute cunt but for some reason I just can't let go of her. There are times when I think that we can get along but every single time she lets me down, makes me the problem or sets me up in some way."

"What about your father?"

"I love him but he's weak. We were very close when I was a kid. I was Daddy's girl and Annie hated it."

"Annie?"

"My mother. My dad took me to see a musical without her once and she freaked out. I remember getting home after an amazing night out and she just tore into my father, telling him that he was rude and disrespectful for not including her. She didn't even ask me if I'd enjoyed it. She just sent me to my room as if I had done something wrong. I'll never, ever, ever forgive her for that."

"And you still want a relationship with her?"

"She's a cunt but she's my mother." It was odd that a seemingly innocuous event such as this had affected her so deeply and remained so vivid in her memory. I wondered whether this had been the beginning of the breakdown of her relationship with her mother.

"Why do you call your mother Annie?"

"She lost the right to be called mother a long time ago." She started pulling at her hair again, drawing the strands between her fingers and thumbs with such force that some of her hair began falling to the ground. "I need to know what's wrong with me." She stopped short, clearly shocked and embarrassed by her own admission.

"*Is* there something wrong with you?"

Martha sat perfectly still, transfixed, and then drew a sharp breath through the corner of her mouth. "According to Annie, *everything's* wrong with me. I'm the black sheep of her shitty little family and everything I've ever done in my life is an insult to her. I got pregnant after a one-night stand, I'm an alcoholic and I refuse to speak to my siblings. I'm everything she doesn't like. She punishes me by trying to drive a wedge between me and my father and he's too weak to stand up to her and defend me."

"But, Martha, with all respect, you're in your sixties. Do you really need to have a relationship with her if it's that bad?" Martha started gripping and squeezing her arms as if she were trying to rid herself of something crawling under her skin. As she did so, I suddenly caught her odour. Throughout our interaction, I had been quietly noting the sensory signals that would lead me to make a diagnosis. The first thing I had noticed was the colour to the side of her eyes – a solid white, like marble. Then there was the sound of her voice, which was reminiscent of someone gently sobbing. Lastly, there was the feeling of loss and longing, an all-pervading grief that filled the room. I had three legs of the stool and now here was the fourth: a rotten odour, not dissimilar to that of an emptied rubbish bin. The smell of decay. My diagnosis was complete. All four sensory signals were telling me that Metal was the causal element and it was clear from her demeanour that it was the Large Intestine official above all that was failing to carry out its remit to remove the waste from body, mind and spirit.

WELCOME FRAGRANCE

"OK, Martha, I've got what I need. Please take off your shoes and make yourself comfortable on the treatment couch. I'm just going to wash my hands." When I came back, the wind outside suddenly picked up, sending a gust of air into the room, and I could hear the gentle pitter-patter of the raindrops as they began falling onto the skylights above. Martha was lying on her back with her eyes closed, her alabaster complexion reminiscent of a lost soul laid to rest.

* * *

Listening to the constant stream of negativity that gushed from Martha's mouth was unsettling. She seemed incapable of looking at her present or past with anything other than disgust and damnation, and her attempts to force the relationship with her mother into a good place felt futile. It led me to think about my own relationships and the relative ease with which I have been able to deal with loss and change. Like most people, I have lost friends and family and while I miss them, I am able to hold them in my heart without suffering the lingering sorrow that so many people experience. Change is not something that I find disruptive. On the contrary, I welcome the chance to move on when my relationship with something or someone feels like it has run its course. The five elements exist as part of a cycle of creation *and* destruction. The Metal element has a key role in this cycle, qualitatively evaluating each and every experience in order to retain only that which is of value. Everything else is discarded.

On an emotional level, the word for this process is forgiveness, the capacity to let go of resentment and anger towards ourselves or others. When I feel hurt or betrayed by someone, I can all too easily send them into exile, so to speak, but the possibility of forgiveness is always there. For those with an imbalance in the Metal element, there's little or no room for forgiveness once the guillotine has dropped. Martha yearned to have a connection with her mother, to be loved and respected by her, but her anger and resentment seemed to have destroyed any chance of a healthy relationship.

The next time I saw Martha she was leaning on the reception desk chatting with Eszter, who grabbed me by the arm as I entered the room.

"Gerad, did you know Martha has a little grey Schnauzer at home? You should tell her to bring him in one day."

Martha pursed her lips and flared her nostrils as if she'd just smelled something bad. "There's no way I'm bringing him in here. He's old, grouchy and incontinent. All he does is drag himself around the house sniffing me. It's disgusting." Eszter and I laughed. It was the first time I had felt light and playful in Martha's presence. I led her downstairs, and as soon as she entered my treatment room, she walked over to the table beside the treatment couch and picked up one of the needles which was still in its packaging. "Can I open it?"

"Be my guest."

She removed the needle from the packet and held it up towards the skylight. "It's so thin. It's amazing what you can do with such a tiny sliver of metal." She sat down in the chair opposite me and began tapping the surface of her hand with the needle. "I felt great after the first treatment."

"In what way?"

"I felt six inches taller. I could *breathe*. Didn't last, though. I got home to find that my son had made a disgusting mess in the kitchen. He's fat and lazy. Treats my flat like a shithole."

"Are you going to say something to him?"

"No need. He won't be coming back. I threw his clothes into a suitcase and sent it round to his brother's house in a taxi."

Rather than react, I chose to say nothing and see what she would do with the silence. She sat still for a few moments, staring into space, and then resumed the frantic tapping of her hand with the needle. Spots of blood appeared in the middle of her palm but she didn't flinch. I couldn't help feeling that she was hurting herself in a desperate attempt to feel something. It was a surprisingly graphic illustration of just how lost and disconnected she was from her body, mind and spirit.

"How *is* your son? You mentioned that he had just broken up from his partner?"

Once again, she looked up and stared for several seconds before the connection was restored. "Both my sons are obese and I mean *obese*. But what can I do? I'm their mum." The manner in which she spoke about her sons felt cold and brutal, yet it seemed to me that some of her anger was directed at herself. As disappointed as she appeared to be in her sons, I had a strong sense that she felt responsible for the way they were, or rather the way she perceived them to be.

"It must have been hard bringing up twins on your own."

"Very hard. I was working full-time, you know? Luckily I was able to work from home but the constant crying and vying for attention drove me insane. Needless to say, Annie never offered to help. She just went on and on about how I should find the father and get some money from him."

"Did you?"

"I couldn't! I have no idea who he was. I remember going to a bar and hooking up with someone but the rest is a blur. I must have blacked out."

When Martha finished speaking, I was left with a slightly empty feeling. It wasn't that her story was uninteresting but the way she told it felt soulless. The words fell out of her mouth as if she were sobbing and there was a distinct lack of poignancy or, indeed, of anything remotely optimistic.

In the West, the popular understanding of what it is to be human is diametrically opposed to that of the ancient Chinese. Westerners tend to believe that we are flesh and blood beings seeking spiritual enlightenment. For the Taoists, the belief is that we are spiritual beings having a human experience. Life is seen through the lens of the five elements and it is the Metal element that keeps us connected to spirit even while we are navigating the dark and murky aspects of this earthly existence. Martha's lifelong struggle to stay connected to her spiritual root meant that all of her attention had been focused on her corporeal existence and the beauty and purity of life had been twisted and bent by the negative and pessimistic lens through which she saw herself and others.

'Soul Door' is a point on the Bladder meridian, located on the upper back, but it has a very close relationship with the Metal element. The Taoists believed that spiritual consciousness only becomes tangible when it incarnates within us. This particular embodiment of the Tao is what we call our 'soul', a unique manifestation of spirit. This spiritual root gives us a profound sense of being connected to the source of life, but it also gives us autonomy and agency in our lives. 'Soul Door' is the doorway for spirit to enter our being, confirming and validating our place in life. I asked Martha to sit up with her legs over the side of the treatment couch and started moulding a small clump of moxa into the shape of a pyramid. She was restless and distracted, pulling at her hair and scratching the back of her neck as she looked from side to side. I warmed the point with seven burning moxa and then inserted the needle through the surface of the skin. As soon as it reached the depth of the acupuncture point, I felt a pull on the needle. I turned it one hundred and eighty degrees clockwise to activate the energy and then withdrew it before placing my finger over the surface of the skin to seal the point. Martha slumped forward. Tears began rolling down her cheeks and her nose began to run. She lay down on the bed and I took the pulses to see if anything had changed. The balance was significantly improved but I needed something more to ground the treatment. 'Meridian Gutter', found on the Lung meridian, acts like a brush to clear the meridians of detritus and make space to receive the pure energy from the heavens. 'Warm Current' on the Large Intestine meridian activates the naturally occurring warmth that emanates from the hidden riches that are locked within. I stood by her side and took the pulses again. The distribution of energy was altogether more balanced and there was greater harmonisation of her colour, sound, odour and emotion.

* * *

The following week, I was on my way back from lunch when my eyes were drawn to a woman gracefully climbing the steps that led to the clinic. There was something mesmerising about the way she was carrying herself, a fluid and confident movement that suggested clarity of purpose and a strong sense of self. As she reached the top of the steps, she turned to look at something in the distance and it was then that I realised it was Martha. It occurred to me that she must be feeling better, but when she walked into my treatment room a few minutes later, she threw her coat on the floor and started pacing around the room as if she had just come home after a bad day.

"What's going on, Martha?"

"I feel awful. I had the whole week planned out – work meetings, AA meetings, helping Uncle Tony – but it's been a complete disaster. I spent the whole week crying."

"When you say awful, can you give me a better sense of what that means for you?"

Martha looked at me in an uncharacteristically clear and alert way. "It's a feeling of emptiness and darkness. I've felt like this on and off for most of my life but this is extreme. It feels like something terrible is about to happen."

I was perplexed. The feeling she described was the exact opposite of what I was experiencing in the room. Her body language was confident, her voice was strong and, most importantly, the connection between us was crystal clear. There was no sign of the vacant stare that had been so noticeable during our first meeting.

"Is it possible, Martha, that despite everything you've told me, you're actually OK beneath it all?"

"What? I feel like shit!"

"Martha, I'm very aware that you've had a challenging time for many years with little or no support but I don't get the sense that you've had the time or space to acknowledge everything you've been through."

Rather than dismiss what I had said, she closed her eyes and nodded. "'Expectations are resentments under construction.' Do you know that saying, Gerad? It never really made sense before but I think I'm starting to get it now. Maybe you're right about me. Normally, I feel so disappointed by everything and everyone but somehow this past week, despite feeling shitty, I've been able to let it all go. It's like I can't be bothered with the drama any more. I also started to question the idea that my life should have been different. I started feeling sorry for myself, too.

That's a first." Martha was calmer and there was even the faintest suggestion of a smile as she stepped back from the drama of the previous week and allowed herself to see it from a place of objectivity. By the end of our discussion, it was clear that Martha's dark night of the soul was in fact a process of truly letting go. It felt like the beginning of something new. In order to reinforce the reactivation of this natural process of elimination, I chose a point called 'Support and Rush Out'. This point is found on the side of the neck, near the end of the Large Intestine meridian. The name of this point tells us that if we are to let go of the things that we no longer need at any given point in our life journey, we need support. The Chinese character for this point depicts the lungs with a chimney stack above. It tells us that the Lung official can hold onto emotions for as long as they are needed, but as soon as they cease to serve a purpose they must be released. This was Martha's opportunity to free herself of everything that was holding her back. When the treatment was finished, she got to her feet and began moving with the same ease and grace with which I had seen her enter the building. I was curious to see if the story of the previous week was still lingering in her head.

"What have you got planned this evening, Martha?"

"Not sure, really. Maybe I'll drop in to see Uncle Tony. We always have a laugh." Just as she was about to leave my room, her phone lit up. "Oh my God! Oh my God! Shit! Shit! Shit!" She grabbed her coat from the back of the door and rushed up the stairs without saying goodbye.

* * *

I emailed Martha to ask if everything was OK but heard nothing back. The following morning, as I was walking my dogs in Regent's Park, my friend Richard called.

"Sorry to hit you with bad news first thing in the morning but there's something I thought I should tell you. Martha's uncle dropped dead yesterday. The cleaner found him lying on the floor in his flat. Martha is devastated."

I left Martha a voice message to express my condolences and offer her whatever help she might need. A few days later, she booked in to see me. She seemed calm but her shoulders were hunched and the blank stare had returned.

"How are you coping, Martha?"

"It's horrible. I miss him so much. I've seen him almost every week of my life and now he's gone."

"What about your mother? Tony was her brother, no?"

"Oh, she's playing the grieving sister. She barely spoke to him for years and now all of a sudden she's acting as if they were best friends. Very convenient. The truth is she despised him because he was gay. I went to see her yesterday and all she could talk about was the inheritance. Uncle Tony didn't leave a will so she gets the lot, apparently. I'll have to contest it. I mean, I'm the one who's looked after him all these years. It's just not fair." I couldn't help thinking how strange it was, knowing how she felt about her mother, that she would have gone to grieve with her and expected anything other than to leave feeling disappointed and resentful.

"Martha, I realise you need to grieve together as a family, but is it good for you to be around your mother if she upsets you so much?"

"She's my mother! I need her to understand how much I did for him. I need her to acknowledge my loss."

"Do you think she's capable of that?"

"I don't know but I'm not giving up."

* * *

Martha disappeared for a few weeks and when she returned she seemed more hurt and angry than ever. "Annie has decided to give everything to the grandchildren. She took such pleasure in telling me. She knew how much it would hurt." Martha was boiling with rage, but the underlying atmosphere in the room was one of deep loss and a profound sense of loneliness and isolation. "I always assumed that he would look after me, you know? I know I had no right to expect anything but I was counting on it. I thought I would finally be able to buy my own home."

As I watched Martha wrestling with her pain and fury, I thought of those old silent movies in which the heroine desperately battles her demons. She was at an important crossroads now. Whatever choice she made would significantly determine the course of her future. Would she pile on yet more layers of anger and resentment or rise above it and start afresh? And what could I do to help her?

'Welcome Fragrance' is the very last point on the Large Intestine meridian, located at the base of the nostrils. It strengthens our natural capacity to free ourselves from the shackles of negativity by rising above the accumulation of decay in body, mind and spirit. Instead, it shifts our focus to the freshness and beauty of the new. Throughout her life, Martha had been consumed by rancour and resentment. It was vital that she finally drag herself out of the noxious pit of fury and cynicism and begin to see her life through a different and altogether more positive lens.

To support and complement 'Welcome Fragrance' I chose 'Head Above Clouds', the second point on the Lung meridian located on the upper chest. This point helps us to rise above the dark clouds of our existence and reconnect with the source. Whenever I take a flight, I feel a sense of elation the moment the plane rises above the clouds to reveal the radiant sunlight and the endless space that surrounds our planet. It's easy to forget that we are part of an infinite, eternal universe when we find ourselves trapped beneath a canopy of clouds. That feeling of isolation and entrapment is, in a metaphorical sense, what those with an imbalance in the Metal element experience throughout their lives. How hard it must be, how alienating, to feel so disconnected from the universe with its limitless potential and freedom.

Each time the needle connected with the point, Martha sighed and then moistened her lips with her tongue. These seemingly trivial signals can often be very significant and are usually far more reliable indicators of change than whatever the patient may be able to articulate in words. To me they felt like gestures of gratitude, silent acknowledgements that this was exactly what she needed. Something changed in Martha that day. After she had put her coat on, she walked over to me and kissed me on both cheeks. This was the first time she had shown any kind of warmth. A gesture of affection is always pleasant to receive but for me it was more than that. As odd as it may seem, I took it as a clear sign from the officials that we were on the right track.

Like all of the seasons, autumn brings a unique quality and designated action. It is the time when Nature breaks everything down and dispenses with anything that it doesn't need to kickstart the next cycle of growth and renewal. It also ensures that the most valuable qualities accumulated during the current cycle are retained and handed down to the Water element for storage. When the Metal element is balanced, this process is effortless. This can be clearly observed in the way that we breathe when our body is functioning at its best. Any imbalance, however, can produce a variety of reactions and symptoms. In Martha's case, her ability to let go of whatever she no longer needed was well and truly compromised. An accumulation of negative thoughts, destructive feelings, obsolete possessions and inappropriate relationships had long held her back from realising her authentic self.

None of us have perfect lives. For starters, we don't get to choose our parents but we *can* choose to what extent we allow them to influence our lives. The same can be said about friendships that lose their quality over time. It is down to us to know when to let people into our lives and when to let them go, and for that we need to tap into the innate intelligence and wisdom of the Metal element. The Large Intestine official embodies the virtue of righteousness and gives us the strength and conviction that we need to stand our ground when others are behaving inappropriately towards us. It gives us the sense that we are of value. When this official is functioning as it should, we are able to take swift and meaningful action when needed, even if it may seem harsh to those around us. Martha's lack of self-worth, combined with her need for the approval of others, in particular her mother, had kept her locked in a dysfunctional victim state that served only to erode whatever traces of self-respect remained.

* * *

When Martha returned the following week, the first thing that caught my attention was her eyes. On our first meeting they had been dull and lifeless but now there was a depth and luminosity about them. She seemed more at ease, too. Although there was still a latent heaviness about her, the signs of change were clear. Apparently, I wasn't the only one to have noticed.

"I think the treatments are working. I can feel the shift."

"I'm happy to hear that, Martha. What's changed?"

"My mother called at the weekend to tell me about the music she had chosen for Uncle Tony's funeral, even though I had already told her what he wanted. Normally I would have gone head-to-head with her. Instead, I just calmly told her that it was not in line with his wishes but that she should do whatever made her happy."

"How did she react?"

Martha broke into a smile. "She didn't react at all. In fact, I realised that she didn't even register what I was saying. All these years I've assumed that she was deliberately ignoring me when actually she probably never heard a single thing I said. You know what I've finally realised?"

"Tell me."

"I mistook my mother for a friend." As Martha continued talking about her week, there was a rare feeling of serenity about her. The sound in her voice was gentler and there was none of the habitual carping and complaining.

"What about the inheritance? Have you come to terms with the loss of your dream?"

"I still think it's unfair and it's hard for me to forgive my mother but I know that there's nothing I can do about it. I've got no choice but to let it go and move on. I'm in my sixties now. I've worked hard all of my life, raised two boys and recovered from a serious addiction. And I've done it all on my own. I'll just have to keep going and make sure I have enough for the future."

The way Martha framed her situation seemed so simple. A pat on the back for what she had achieved and recognition that she needed to secure her future. Could it really be that simple? The contrast of embattled, resentful Martha with philosophical, forward-looking Martha was testament to the power of the Metal element when it cuts down the weeds, clears the path and makes way for something new.

Martha committed to weekly treatment for the next two months. I explained that although she had experienced a breakthrough, she should not expect a miracle. The process of letting go and grieving takes time, whatever form the loss may take. People, things, behaviours, attitudes – all of them need to be released little by little. Over the following weeks, this cautionary strategy worked well as she was repeatedly challenged by family dynamics around the death of her uncle. Her sister, whose three young daughters were in line to inherit a substantial sum of money, wrote to Martha asking her never to mention that Uncle Tony was a "poof". Martha was furious, but instead of flying off the handle she managed to contain her anger and simply resolved to tell her nieces about Uncle Tony's sexuality as soon as they were old enough to understand. Anything less would have been dishonourable and disrespectful, she told me.

Much like the unsung heroes who sift through our rubbish and extract whatever can be recycled, the Large Intestine official has a thankless but vital task. It is the expert in identifying and removing waste in order to preserve the health of our body, mind and spirit. Martha underwent a gradual but pronounced transformation over the following months. Her lightness of being could be seen in every aspect of her physical, mental and spiritual health. She looked brighter, carried herself with greater ease and embraced life with an altogether more positive attitude. It was a far cry from the harsh and vengeful person that I had first encountered. It turned out that Uncle Tony had left a will after all. He had posted it to himself a year before his death and Martha's nephew had found it in a drawer full of unopened letters while they were clearing out his flat. He had left half of his estate to Martha and the other half to his great-nephews and

-nieces. Martha was thrilled that she would finally be able to buy her own home but, remarkably, she took the news of the inheritance in her stride. It seemed that she no longer needed material gain or external validation in order to feel happy.

5

LISTENING PALACE

*

Jack dropped into the armchair and grinned at me. "Before we get going, there's something you need to know about me. I'm a wealthy man." I blinked and shook my head, the way you do when someone says something completely random.

"OK, Jack. I'll bear that in mind." I often tell my students that if you remain alert from the very first moment a new patient walks into the room, they will tell you everything you need to know. Jack's opening salvo sounded straightforward enough, but it was also jarring, as was his outfit, which was a peculiar hybrid of Midwestern cowboy and Bohemian chic.

"Let's face it, G, when you meet someone for the first time you just want to stick your head in the oven and end it all." I had no idea what he was talking about but I couldn't help smiling. "Do you mind if I call you 'G'? I can't get my head round your name. It's missing a letter." He took off his hat and started spinning it on his finger.

"Whatever works for you, Jack. Now, I'm just going to

give you my treatment preamble so that you understand the process."

"Hold on a second. Check this out!" He grabbed his coat from the floor beside his chair and removed two sponge balls from one of the pockets. "Hold your hands out, G. Palms up." He placed one of the balls in my left hand and told me to close my fists as tightly as possible. He then placed the other ball in his own hand and did the same. "Right, open your hands, G." The ball had disappeared. "Abracadabra, baby!" He opened his hands and two balls dropped to the floor. He giggled with delight and rocked in his chair, lifting both his feet off the ground. "Don't you just love that, man?" The twinkle in his eyes was mesmerising, but I felt like I was losing control of my practice space.

"Right! Back to business, Jack. I need to go through what we…" Before I could finish my sentence, Jack was on the floor, manoeuvring himself into a backbend. "This is the camel pose. Been doing yoga since my early twenties. It's my spiritual calling, man. This is about as far as I can go. Any further and my lower back gives out."

"Jack, can we get started, please? Let's talk about why you're here." He unravelled himself, jumped to his feet and did a star jump before settling back into the chair.

"Is that why you're here, Jack, for your back pain?"

"No. I'm here because I'm struggling to manifest the wealth I deserve in my life. I feel like I'm doing all the right things but the universe isn't showing up. There's friction, man." I dropped my file to the floor. There was clearly no point making notes.

LISTENING PALACE

* * *

The first time I saw Jack was on a bitterly cold day in mid-February. I was sitting in a local coffee shop when the door swung open and a tall man with shoulder-length hair burst in like a gust of wind. He was wearing a long suede coat with a shaggy collar, bright red corduroy shorts and cowboy boots. The moment he walked in, the atmosphere in the shop changed. He grabbed a baguette from the shelf and started tearing pieces off with his mouth while he queued for his coffee. When it was his turn to order, he called the barista "baby" and started juggling with some tangerines, which he had plucked from a basket by the counter. Everyone was looking at him and he knew it. Once his cappuccino was ready, he stuffed the remainder of the baguette into his pocket, doffed his hat to the room and disappeared into the street without closing the door behind him. It was the most bizarre spectacle, at once amusing and disturbing. I never imagined that this man would soon be bringing that same startling and disruptive energy into my clinic, but here he was.

"What does manifesting wealth in your life mean to you, Jack?"

"Money! I'm a financial advisor and I manage a large portfolio of clients. Drawing down abundance is what I'm known for. It's my mission in life. My clients consider what I bring to them to be virtual fixed assets." He looked confused, as if the words that came out of his mouth had been spoken by someone else. I was also confused.

"I must confess this is not an area I'm familiar with, so

forgive me if I don't quite understand what you're talking about."

"I can't help you there, G. My relationship with my clients is confidential."

"I see." I didn't see, but I was keen to move on to something that made sense. "Jack, could you give me a bit of your personal history? What was your childhood like?"

"We had a big problem with emetophobia in our household. My sisters lived in a permanent state of fear and sometimes they couldn't even go to school."

"I'm sorry, Jack, what do you mean?"

"It was the bulimia."

"Your sisters had bulimia?"

"No, Deirdre did."

"Deirdre?"

"My aunt. She used to stay with us for weeks on end."

"So your sisters had a fear of vomiting and your aunt would come to the house and make herself throw up?"

"Exactly. It was very troubling." Talking to him was exhausting. It felt like he was tossing pieces of a puzzle at me and expecting me to put them together in real time. I eventually gathered that he had been born in Manchester, and was one of three children. His parents were both teachers in the local state school but he and his sisters had been educated privately.

"Why was that, Jack? Didn't your parents think a state education would be good enough?"

"They were dead proud of their school. Top notch, man. But they wanted us to go to a private school. It wasn't as good as their school but at the same time it was better, so yeah, you know, swings and roundabouts. It's a prestige thing." My head was spinning. "You see, if I hadn't been to private school, I wouldn't have met the kind of people that I needed to build my financial empire. It's who you know, you know? Gotta be able to move in different circles and blend in." I started to feel a knot in my stomach. Everything about him felt chaotic, just as it had that day in the coffee shop. The idea that he could "blend in" was laughable. He was like a cat in a room full of pigeons.

* * *

"That which takes charge of the Being is called the Heart." This quote, taken from the Huangdi Neijing, an ancient text on Chinese medicine, tells us that it is not the mind that controls our lives, but rather the heart. With its integral relationship to the source of life, the Heart official maintains a sense of control and order over all the other Officials by its presence alone. It's the same concept as a figurehead who exerts a benign influence over a domain without actually exercising power. In order to maintain peace and order, the Heart must maintain its authority in the face of continual disturbances and threats from within and without. It can only do this with the assistance of its partner, the Small Intestine. In Western terms, the small intestine is just one part of the long and complex digestive system, but we should not underestimate the importance of what it does. When we eat something, the food passes first of all into the stomach, where it is broken down and turned into a digestive mix known as chyme. The stomach then passes the chyme to the small intestine, where an intricate process of sorting takes place, courtesy of hundreds of billions of tiny finger-like projections called microvilli. Anything that is beneficial to our being is absorbed into the body for energy. Anything that is injurious is sent down to the large intestine for excretion. The small intestine knows exactly what we need at any given moment and the choices it makes vary accordingly. From a Western perspective, this is what maintains our physical wellbeing. For the Chinese, this ability to sort the pure from the impure applies to body, mind and spirit alike. All of the organs, or officials, reside within one of the five elements. In the case of the Small Intestine official, it is the Fire element. This official is paired with the Heart and between them they govern and maintain the propriety and purity of our existence. In simple terms, we live in a world that is composed of pure and impure (good and bad) and therefore we need a system that can discriminate between the two and maintain the correct balance.

* * *

The absence of any coherent thread in Jack's account of his life was thoroughly disorienting, so I started drawing pictures in an attempt to make sense of what he was telling me. Before long, the page on my clipboard was covered in doodles, connected by a network of circles and arrows that tried in vain to tie everything together.

"Help me out here, Jack, why do you need four different storage units?"

"Because both of my parents are dead."

"So… you're storing their possessions, too?"

"Exactly. In Manchester. But every now and again I take a carload to the storage unit in Essex."

"Oh, I see, you're planning to sell it."

"Why would I do that? I told you, it's my parents' stuff." After the initial burst of party tricks and laughter, Jack seemed to be rapidly losing steam and had become rather flat and serious. It felt as if his fire had burned out and all that was left was a small blue flame, flickering in the embers.

When I see a patient for the first time, I normally spend at least an hour gathering information, but with Jack it was clearly a futile endeavour. My questions seemed to bore him, and I had the sense that he disliked being in the spotlight unless it was his show. In any case, despite – or perhaps because of – our rather bizarre first interaction, I felt that I already had enough to make a diagnosis. The colour in his face, especially around the temples, was ashen, and the scorched odour that he gave off was so strong that I had initially wondered if he was a smoker. Both of these were telltale signs of an imbalance in the Fire element. The other two distinguishing features that I needed to make a full diagnosis – sound and emotion – were also clearly identifiable. When he wasn't playing the clown, the feeling that remained was a profound lack of joy and the timbre of his voice was correspondingly flat and lifeless. Nature was telling me to reinvigorate the Fire.

THE UNTAPPED SELF

The stimulation of this causal element would naturally set off a chain reaction of controlled regeneration: the Fire creating the Earth, the Earth creating the Metal, the Metal creating the Water, the Water creating the Wood, the Wood creating the Fire. Within the Fire element, the focus of treatment would be the Small Intestine official, which was malfunctioning to such a degree that I was nervous to lift the lid on this man's chaotic life. When I did, the mask of the joker soon fell away and I began to see a different, altogether more toxic side to him.

"How old are you, Jack?" I asked him as I wrapped up the questions.

"Old enough to know that I never want to sleep with a woman over twenty-five again." He must have seen me wince because he immediately jumped to his feet and did a little shimmy. "Let's get to it! If you ask any more questions we'll have nothing to talk about next time." At the end of the treatment, as he was gathering up his things, I took out my card machine to take payment. He stopped what he was doing and gave me a cold stare.

"I don't do cards, man. I'll pay you for six sessions upfront. Cash. I'll bring it with me next time, OK? Thanks, G, it's been real." Before I could say anything, he was off, leaping up the stairs two at a time.

* * *

Hello Jack,
It was great to meet you today. I hope you're feeling well from the treatment. I just wanted to remind you of our

payment terms as outlined in previous correspondence. Payment can be made by cash or card and must be paid at the point of service. We require 48 hours' notice for cancellation or changes to booked appointments.
 I look forward to seeing you next week.
 Best wishes
 Gerad

Hey G!
Thanks for the needles. Feeling great!!! I'm going to open a trade account for you with one of my offshore companies which pays 8% interest. I'll sign up on your behalf and add £2k to your new account to cover the first 10 treatments. My runner will deliver your interest payments monthly in cash. Send me your full name, passport number and address and I'll get it all set up. Great doing business with you, man.
 Jack

* * *

On a particularly gloomy day in June, I arrived at the clinic to find Eszter looking somewhat flustered. "What's going on, Eszter? You've got glitter on your face." She blushed and mouthed something.

"What?"

"Shh!" She motioned towards the waiting room. "Mid-night-Cow-boy." I walked into the room and found Jack slumped in one of the armchairs. His hat was tipped forward over his face and he was snoring. There was a feather boa round his neck and his face was speckled with purple glitter. He looked like he had just walked out of a night club.

"Good morning, Jack." Jack jolted out of his slumber and raised his hat to reveal a pair of aviator sunglasses, which he pushed up the bridge of his nose before flicking me a 'V' sign. "Peace, brother. What took you so long?"

"You do know you're an hour early, right?"

"Nice try, G! Love your sense of humour." I pulled out my phone and scrolled through my emails.

"There you go, Jack." He winked and pulled down his hat. "No worries. I'll take a nap." My job as an 'instrument of Nature' is to pay attention to what I'm experiencing through my senses and steer clear of mental judgements. Jack was such an interesting and colourful character that it was hard not to be seduced by the show. Nevertheless, it was essential for me to remain focused if I wanted to uncover what he truly needed.

After I had finished with my next patient, I buzzed Eszter and asked her to send Jack down while I went to wash my hands. When I walked back into the room, he was sitting in the armchair in the lotus position with his eyes closed

"Did you have a good rest?"

"Yeah, all good, man. I felt great after your treatment, by the way. Full of energy. I could feel the flow."

"Is there anything else you've noticed?"

"Yeah. Your receptionist. Way too old for me but I bet she was a cracker in her day."

"What have you noticed about *yourself*, Jack?"

"G! You're too serious, man. OK, what have I noticed? Well, I'm dialling up a lot more business and I've taken on Little Erik full-time."

"Little Erik?"

"My runner."

"Oh yes, you mentioned him in your email. We need to talk about that at the end of the session."

"Nothing to talk about, G. It's simple. I keep all my clients topped up with the interest on their investments, so Little Erik is a busy boy on his scooter whizzing around town keeping everyone happy. You'll love him. He's like me but about half the size."

The word that kept popping into my head was 'shady', yet the allure of this man was irresistible. I felt like I was being sucked into an alternate reality where nothing made sense and the cast of characters got stranger by the second. I was almost tempted to agree to his 'deal' just so that I could meet Little Erik.

"I'm happy to hear that your business has picked up. What do you put that down to? My treatment?" I was intrigued to know what he would do with my joke, but rather than take the bait he leaned forward and locked eyes with me.

"Gloria Eisner has just signed up to my investment bundle. She's planning one of her Mahjong nights so she can introduce me to some of her circle. Smart lady. Knows a good opportunity when she sees one. You should take a leaf out of her book."

"Well, I have no idea who Gloria Eisner is, but I will certainly bear it in mind if I have some spare cash." Jack began to tell me about his home life. He claimed that he lived in a penthouse apartment in Notting Hill with his girlfriend of fifteen years. He drove a Range Rover, threw extravagant parties for his clients and took regular breaks in their villa in Ibiza. He also told me that someone was spying on him.

"Really? What makes you think that?" He handed me his phone on which there was a grainy image of what looked like dimly lit trees. I had a sudden urge to burst out laughing but I restrained myself.

"Jack, that sounds scary. Can you tell me more?"

"I'm a successful man, Gerad. There are people out there who want to bring me down."

The atmosphere in the room had suddenly changed. I no longer felt the levity. In its place was something rather dark and menacing. Furthermore, I had lost control of the interaction. I sat upright and tried to reassert my authority, but he was already back in the driving seat.

"You don't mind, do you?" Jack had taken a bag of tobacco from his pocket and was busy rolling a cigarette.

"You can't smoke in here, Jack."

"Why not? You smoke weed all the time. I can smell it from the street."

"That's moxa, Jack. It's a Chinese herb. And I don't smoke it. I burn it to warm up the acupuncture point before I needle it."

"Not the most convincing story, G. 'Your honour, I had no idea the truck was full of weed. It was supposed to be a shipment of Chinese herbs.'" Our interaction had now morphed into a kind of playful bickering, but as inappropriate as it was, it felt impossible to break out of it.

"Jack, please."

He winked at me. "I'm kidding, man. I'm rolling it for when I leave. Talking about stuff makes me nervous." I was starting to understand the way Jack operated. He had a way of undermining my authority in the room by switching personas and throwing me off balance. I felt manipulated, and given that I was the person charged with helping him, it was not a healthy dynamic.

"OK, Jack, on the couch, please. I need to treat you now. Down to your underpants, please, and pull the blanket over you." Jack removed his brightly coloured hippie trousers and vaulted onto the treatment couch as if he were doing the high jump.

"Do your worst, G!"

From a diagnostic and treatment perspective, I was dealing with a Fire that was unstable and unpredictable. Restoring the healthy functionality of the Fire element with needles is every bit as challenging as building and managing a real fire. Having already made contact with the Fire officials in my first treatment, my next line of action was to ensure that the Wood element, which is the mother of the Fire element, was available to feed her child. I chose two points on the Heart and Small Intestine channels that naturally attract the Wood to the Fire. Towards the end of the treatment, despite a marked change for the better in him, I began to feel anxious as I knew I would have to speak to Jack about my payment terms. It was simple enough. He was required to pay at the end of each session just like everyone else, but for some reason I was reluctant to confront him. After I had finished taking the pulses, Jack slid off the table, pulled on his trousers and excused himself. Two minutes later, I heard the sound of the toilet flushing and then a familiar voice outside my door.

"Gotta run, G! Don't forget to send me your passport number."

I was being played.

* * *

Jack cancelled his third appointment and I decided not to chase him for the payment. The two sessions I had had with him, while memorable, had been challenging, and I was keen to put the whole thing down to experience and move on. Then, a few months later, I heard something unexpected, yet somehow unsurprising. I had just returned from my lunch break one day when Eszter beckoned me over to her desk.

"Gerad! Do you know Gloria Eisner?"

"The name rings a bell. Why?"

"She was just here to see the dentist upstairs. She told me that Midnight Cowboy has been arrested."

"Jack? Arrested? For what?"

"Fraud. Gloria met him in the waiting room and he roped her into a Ponzi scheme. The whole thing was a scam."

* * *

Over the next few years, I barely thought about Jack, but then one morning, I switched on my laptop and found an email from him.

G!
Long time no see. Sorry for the disappearing act. I got myself into a bit of trouble and I've been living at Her Majesty's pleasure for the past three years. I'll fill you in when I see you. Anyway, I'm back. Can I book in for a tune-up?
Jack x

I was enjoying a rare moment of quiet when Eszter appeared in the doorway looking unusually excited.
"Is everything alright, Eszter?"
"He's back!"
"Who's back?"
"Jack's back!"
I looked at my schedule for the day. "You're right. I'd forgotten it was today. I'll be up shortly, OK?" The thought of seeing Jack again made me nervous. Instead of going up to meet him right away, I started finding things to do. Was I trying to let him know who was in control by making him wait? Or was I simply nervous to be in the company of this unpredictable man once again? I had agreed to see him knowing full well about his recent spell in prison and in spite of the overdue payments, so there was clearly still something to be learned from this relationship, something to be resolved. At ten minutes past the hour, I took a deep breath, climbed the stairs

and walked along the corridor to the waiting room. Jack was standing in front of the fireplace playing with a string of beads. He was dressed in an ankle-length coat made of dozens of brightly coloured patches and a pair of basketball boots with bright blue laces. His hair had been tied into a bun and he had a long beard speckled with patches of grey. I felt as though I was standing in front of a Himalayan guru.

"G! I'd recognise those magical footsteps of yours anywhere. Great to see you, man. I've missed you."

"Great to see you, too, Jack." I was genuinely delighted to see him and more than a little relieved. Since his conviction, I had somewhat demonised him in my mind, but here he was, the larger-than-life character that I had briefly come to know, disarming me once again with his warmth and eccentricity. I led him downstairs and retrieved his file as he hung his technicolour coat on the back of the door.

"Where do we start, Jack? It's been a while." I was expecting to hear a tale of regret and repentance but I was sorely mistaken. No sooner had he settled into the chair than he launched into an impassioned rant against the judicial system and the financial regulators. His conviction had been a terrible miscarriage of justice, he told me, a conspiracy by the metropolitan elites who didn't take kindly to an upstart from Manchester making money on their patch. But it was just a temporary setback. He was preparing to relaunch his business, it would be bigger and better, it was his destiny.

"You know what, G, while I was locked up I had a lot

of time to reflect on how I was living my life."

"It's always good to have time to reflect, Jack. What was the most valuable lesson that you learned?"

"It's simple, G. I need to be clear with stupid people, speak very, very slowly, repeat things, and when I see their little brains struggling to understand me, be patient and understanding."

I was aghast at what I was hearing. I had assumed that he wanted my help to set him on a new path in life, that he would show some humility and contrition. It was naive, to say the least. It appeared that little had changed and he seemed destined to repeat the same pattern of behaviour that had landed him in trouble in the first place.

I had no reason to doubt my original diagnosis, so despite everything that had happened since I last saw him, my focus remained on constructing a treatment plan that would support the Fire element. Anything beyond that was out of my control. The Small Intestine is responsible for sorting every aspect of our lives. It gives us purity of purpose and clarity not only within ourselves but also in how we perceive and interact with the world. When this official is out of balance, problems with control are commonplace, resulting in confusion and chaos. This is by no means to excuse or justify Jack's wrongdoing, but rather to shine a different light on what might have driven him to act in that way. Had Jack been in a state of balance, I believe that he probably would have seen how flawed, indeed how crooked, his scheme was. From my brief experience of him, however, he seemed unable to see anything with clarity, let alone a complex investment structure involving hundreds of people.

Although Jack's demeanour was much the same as before, there was a dullness in his eyes that saddened me, and his effervescence seemed forced. How, I wondered, could the fire be reignited without him losing control and burning down the house again?

"Jack, how exactly can I help you? It's important we have some defined markers so we can gauge if treatment is working for you."

"I just need you on Jack's team, man. That's it."

Jack fascinated me and infuriated me in equal measure but I had to put my personal reactions aside. He had entrusted himself to my care and my responsibility was to stay true to my role.

"Jack, I am happy to help you as best I can, but I need you to commit to a treatment and payment schedule." Jack nodded and thrust his bejewelled hand towards me. The deal was done. He removed his shoes, hopped onto the treatment couch and held his hands together in a gesture of prayer.

"Hit me up, G!"

My starting point with treatment that day was to acknowledge the loss of Jack's greatest asset, the twinkle in his eyes. In Chinese philosophy, this was seen as a lack of 'shen' or spirit. The Huangdi Neijing states that "acupuncture must move the patient's spirit to be successful – it is not merely mechanical". 'Spirit Burial Ground' is a point on the Kidney meridian, located directly over the heart. It is here that the Heart and Kidney officials are united in their purpose of resurrecting our spirit, just as the sun brings life to the oceans. As I warmed the point with moxa, he took a few deep breaths, and immediately after the needle reached the point, his face flooded with warmth. I ended the treatment with two points to support the Fire.

Jack dressed himself, reached into the pocket of his coat and handed me a wad of cash. "That's for three sessions. Plus eight per cent interest." The inimitable twinkle was back.

* * *

Five days later, Jack was back in the chair.

"How are you doing, Jack?"

"I don't understand what's going on, G. I've been reaching out to some of my old mates but they seem to have joined the other side."

"The other side?"

"They keep going on about my old business being dodgy. A couple of them lost money and they want me to pay it back. It's simple, man, the business went bust. I couldn't maintain it. How could I? I was in prison."

According to ancient Chinese philosophy, it is the heart, not the mind, that is the arbiter of truth. When we speak from the heart, it is the Heart official that represents us with a trustworthy voice. Similarly, when we listen to the words of another, it is the Small Intestine official, which is connected to the Heart, that ensures we retain only that which is good and aligns with the truth.

This process of sorting the pure from the impure is not a rational process, nor does it require any effort. It is an automatic filtering system that enables us to enjoy the colour and complexity of this world without straying from the path. If Jack were able to stay connected to the truth, he would undoubtedly find a way to express his bright, exuberant self without falling victim to his darker impulses. Based on these simple but profound principles, I selected two points that would help to reinstate this natural human capacity.

'Utmost Source' is the first point on the Heart meridian and connects directly to the centre of the heart itself. Its function is to keep us connected to the source of life, enabling us to know who we are at the most primal level. Without that relationship, we feel joyless, lost and alone, commonly resulting in a loss of control or, conversely, a tendency to over-control all aspects of our life. The second point was 'Listening Palace'. This is the final point on the Small Intestine meridian, located next to the opening of the ear. Its gift is clarity and discernment. The 'Listening Palace' is the place where we hear "the chimes of heaven", the sound of truth that enables us to differentiate between the purity of heaven and the impure nature of the world that we inhabit. This point filters out anything that would prevent us from fulfilling our destiny with clarity of vision and purpose.

Another week passed, and although I thought the treatment had been precisely what he needed, it was clear that Jack's inner chaos and confusion were still overriding even the most potent interventions.

"There's some kind of conspiracy out there, G. People are coming up with all kinds of stories about me. They're all losers."

"Jack, from what you've told me, people lost money after they invested in your scheme. They are bound to have regrets, don't you think?"

"Abundance comes to those who wear its charms. You know that. You're a successful man. That doesn't come from pandering to gossip."

As usual, Jack wasn't making any sense. I felt I had no choice other than to step in and take control of the situation. While it was not my business to desire or expect a certain outcome, I knew that as long as Jack's Heart and Small Intestine officials were not functioning correctly, things would only get worse. I felt that I owed it to him to up my game and take a calculated risk. The ability to know the truth is a natural capacity that we all possess, but sometimes we become blind to it. Jack's inability to see the criminal nature of his actions, let alone understand the consequences, was a sign of just how disconnected he had become from his authentic self. It prompted me to think about using an acupuncture point on the Small Intestine official, part of a group of points called 'The Windows', which gives us the capacity to see not only with the physical eye, but also with the mental and spiritual eye. However, choosing to use a point such as this early in treatment can be a gamble, because often people need time before they are able to face their truth. Was Jack ready to face up to what he had done? I asked him to turn his head to emphasise the musculature of his neck. The Window of the Small Intestine is found at the back of the muscle that extends from the base of the skull to the sternum. As the needle reached the depth of the point, Jack tensed momentarily and then let out a long, primal howl. He left my treatment room in a very different state that day. Instead of his usual ebullience, he was reserved, gentle and quiet.

* * *

The following week, the man who came to see me was almost unrecognisable as Jack. His head was hung low and his outfit was completely devoid of colour.

"What's going on, Jack? You seem a bit out of sorts."

"I'm not feeling that great, to be fair. Everything's gone a bit weird."

"In what way?"

"After I left here last week, I stopped off at my local pub. I know all the bar staff there but rather than shoot the shit with them, I sat in the corner with my beer. I was completely paranoid."

"Paranoid?"

"It was like being that shy kid in Manchester all over again. I was convinced that everyone was staring and laughing at me. I walked home and went straight to bed."

"How did you feel in the morning?"

"I felt good but everything was really trippy. I started seeing things in my flat that I hadn't noticed before, like the way the floor sloped near the front door. Everything sounded different. The boiler, the clock, the traffic. Everything was amplified." As Jack slowly unpacked his week, he told me every little thing he had noticed about himself and his environment. There was a freshness and an endearing childlike quality to him. It was as if he were exploring the world for the very first time and was eager to share it with me. The change was remarkable.

"Jack, you said you weren't feeling great today but you don't give that impression at all. What's up?"

"I don't know, G. I just feel different. I can't put my finger on it."

Jack continued to come for regular treatment and soon showed a marked improvement on all levels, including – to my great relief – the way he communicated. When he first came to see me, I had struggled to make sense of what he was saying as he meandered from one thought to another with little or no unifying thread. My experience of him was different now. The new Jack seemed grounded and thoughtful, and our interaction felt altogether more balanced and harmonious. To help him to maintain his new-found clarity, I asked him to keep a journal of how he was feeling. A few weeks later, he announced he'd abandoned plans to rebuild his investment business.

"Have you thought about what you'd like to do instead?" I asked him.

"You've forgotten about my spiritual calling, G. I'm going to teach yoga!"

"Of course! Yoga is the perfect fit."

Jack signed up for an intensive teacher training programme, and every time he came to see me he would proudly demonstrate the latest pose that he had perfected. He also began to show a keen interest in my work. As I was treating him, he would ask me to explain what I was doing, think about it for a while, and then carefully rephrase what I had said. It was as if he had passed my words through a filter to refine them or even, on occasions, imbue them with more meaning. I was surprised and fascinated. Had Jack become my teacher?

Six months into treatment, Jack was doing better than I could possibly have hoped, but one day I got an email from him saying that he needed to cancel his next two sessions. There was no apology and no explanation, just an uncharacteristically curt message. When he turned up a fortnight later, he had a glum expression on his face.

"What's the matter, Jack? You look worried."

"G, I don't know how to tell you this."

"Tell me what?"

"I'm going back to prison."

I was stunned. "What happened, Jack?"

"After our last session I suddenly spun out of control." He lowered his head and clasped his hands around the back of his neck.

"Jack?" For a moment he didn't move, but then his shoulders started shaking. He leaned forward in his chair, slapped me on the knee and burst out laughing. "G! Don't look so serious! I'm fucking with you, man! I've landed a gig teaching yoga in a prison. I start next week. And… I'm launching my own studio with someone I met on the teacher training! We've been working flat out for the past two weeks getting it all ready."

Jack's new career went from strength to strength. His charisma and energy attracted a loyal following and it wasn't long before he opened a second studio. The waiting room in my clinic became a recruiting ground for him and several of my patients signed up for his classes. Not only my patients, in fact. One morning I arrived at the clinic to find Eszter rolling up a yoga mat. As soon as she saw me, she pushed it under her desk.

"Why are you looking at me like that, Gerad?"

"It was only a matter of time, Eszter."

* * *

Jack reminded me of Dr Jekyll and Mr Hyde. We all have good and bad as part of our makeup but we get to choose which of those two impulses to embrace. Most of us err on the side of right action. If we do embrace the dark side, it is a conscious choice that we make in full awareness of the possible consequences. For some people, however, the seemingly obvious distinction between good and evil is flipped on its head. This is particularly apparent in criminals whose complex belief system appears to justify manipulation, lying and the violation of rules. From the ancient Chinese perspective, it is the responsibility of the Fire element and its official, the Small Intestine, to set us on the right path. When the Fire is functioning as it should, that path is clearly seen. When it ceases to do so, there is a constant danger that we will lose our way. I don't believe for a minute that Jack meant to harm anyone. He was a joy to be around and the energy that he exuded did not come from a dark place. But within him, confusion reigned. When there was a fair wind, so to speak, the Fire within him burnt in a controlled manner and his spirit shone brightly. When there was an ill wind, however, the Fire would blaze out of control and chaos would ensue.

The Fire element is a creative force – without the sun there would be no life on earth, after all – but it can also destroy. This delicate balance between creation and destruction is a fundamental challenge for humans. We need warmth, passion and love for every aspect of our existence but the source of these qualities must be carefully managed. I am all too aware of this challenge, having been diagnosed many years ago as having an imbalance in the Fire element. Despite decades of supportive acupuncture treatment, there are still times when something happens and my Fire is extinguished. That's when I crave the high to pull me out of my joyless, ashen state, but it's precisely that high that can get me into trouble. Equally, there are times when my passions are aroused so intensely that I struggle to keep them under control. Being with Jack was always exhilarating. To use a well-worn phrase, he lit up the room wherever he went. But as with anyone whose Fire shines so brightly, there was always the risk that it would either die out or burn out of control. Despite his remarkable transformation, there was always a part of me that expected to switch on the news and see him running for office or being led away in handcuffs. Maybe even both.

6

EARTH MOTIVATOR

*

It was late August when George arrived for his first appointment. It was still warm but autumn was waiting in the wings, eager to take centre stage, and the days were beginning to grow shorter. Eszter seemed flustered when she announced George's arrival and I soon found out why. I walked into the waiting room to find a tall, handsome man in his mid-twenties with wavy blonde hair, blue eyes and the physique of an athlete. He was dressed simply in jeans, a linen shirt with the sleeves rolled up and trainers that had traces of dried mud on them. He leapt to his feet to offer me his hand and unveiled a set of perfect white teeth framed by a broad grin. It might have been quite intimidating to be met with such physical perfection, but there was an insecurity about him that immediately made me feel as if I were in the presence of a child. He looked at me with the imploring, wide-eyed expression of a puppy, and instead of being overawed, I felt as though I should be wrapping him in a blanket and reassuring him that everything was going to be OK.

"You must be George," I said, taking his hand.

"Yes, that's right, I'm George." He gripped my hand and shook it vigorously. "What a lovely part of London this is. You're perfectly positioned between two parks. Amazing! I love the parks. I'm a gardener, you know. Well, I say I'm a gardener, actually I've only been doing it for six months and now I'm on gardening leave!" He laughed out loud at his own joke and seemed a little disappointed that I didn't do the same.

"My treatment room is this way, George. Grab your things and I'll take you down there." As I led him down the stairs, he talked incessantly and kept so close to me that we were almost touching. It was as if he were terrified of breaking this newly formed bond. I stood in the doorway and ushered him into my room. As he walked past me, I caught his odour. It was like fermenting beer, sickly sweet and cloying.

"So, George, tell me a bit about yourself. What brings you here?"

"Jessica sent me."

"Yes, I'm aware of that, but is there any particular reason?"

"I screwed up at work. She said she'd give me a second chance if I came for treatment."

"And what about you personally? Is there anything you would like help with?"

"Not really. I mean, I get a bit anxious sometimes, but that's normal, isn't it? Other than that, you know, I have to be careful with what I eat or I get constipated. I take probiotics to keep my microbiome in good shape and I don't touch grains or dairy products. Should I be worried about the constipation? I mean, I can go for tests if you think it's serious." George was sitting on the edge of his chair, leaning towards me with his hands folded in his lap. His body language was submissive and his eyes were moist and blinking. Despite his imposing form, he looked like a child waiting to see the dentist.

"OK, so there are a few things we can look at together, but why don't we start with what happened at work? And by the way, please know that you can talk freely. As you know, Jessica is also a patient of mine, but anything you say in here is confidential."

"It was nothing really. Just a spat with someone I work with. Jessica thought it best that I disappear for a while until things cool down."

"A spat? Can you elaborate?"

George lowered his head like a naughty schoolboy and then all of a sudden he started rubbing his hands together as if he were about to tuck into a plate of his favourite food.

"I've just thought of something else you can help me with!" He leapt to his feet and started tapping on the door with his knuckles. "I have this weird OCD thing. Whenever I leave the house, I have to knock on the door three times, tap my heels together and then spin the keys on my index finger before I lock it. Quite often I don't even make it to the end of the road before I have to go back and check if it's locked."

It was a pretty good swerve but I persisted. "George, come and sit down, please. Compulsive behaviour is something I can help you with but it would be really helpful for me to know what it was that led you to come here in the first place. Why did Jessica ask you to take time off?"

George plonked himself back in the chair and huffed like a moody teenager. "I was getting on just fine and then Jessica went and hired this nasty girl called Lucy who thinks she's a bloke."

"You mean she's a lesbian?"

"Exactly." He made a face and started wringing his hands as if he were trying to get rid of something sticky and annoying. "She's really mean and sarcastic, and whenever I take my shirt off to cool down she whistles at me. I think she's jealous that I actually *am* a man."

He lowered his gaze and continued playing with his hands. His body language was odd, but the thing that really caught my attention was how still he was. Were it not for the movement of his hands, anyone would have thought that he was sitting in meditation. I observed him for a moment in silence, and it suddenly occurred to me how much he resembled one of those heroic sculptures. The muscles in his arms and face were taut and the skin that covered them was completely free of blemishes or any sign of vascularity.

"OK, so there was a bit of friction between you but I'm assuming that wasn't all, am I right?"

"She's very political and she kept going on and on about stuff and asking me what I thought. So irritating. I don't care about that kind of thing, you know?"

"Can you give me an example?"

"She's trying to get elected to the local council and her campaign is woke beyond belief. She wants to open a centre for people who have been queer bashed. I mean, seriously, who cares, right?" He looked at me with pleading eyes, the way my dogs do when they are hoping for some scraps from the table.

"So you'd rather be talking about something more fun while you're digging the garden?" My frivolous comment didn't sit well with him. He sat back in the chair, crossed his arms and furrowed his brow like a child having a tantrum. "George, I'm still struggling to understand why Jessica had to let you go. What did you do that was so bad?"

"Nothing." George was sulking and I had lost my rapport with him. I needed to wind back and see what I had missed.

"I'm sorry, George. It must be really hard having to come here when it's not your own choice and I'm sure you have very good reasons for doing whatever it was you did."

He uncrossed his arms and looked at me with puppy eyes. It was suddenly clear to me that my sympathetic approach had been welcomed with open arms. George was desperate to be heard and understood. Together with the strong odour that I had noticed when he entered the room, these two sensory signals suggested that his causal element might be Earth, but it was too early to jump to any conclusions.

Making sense of our mysterious existence is no easy task, particularly if we try to do it alone. Fortunately, there are countless others with whom we can share the experience of being human for our mutual benefit. This is called reciprocity. The natural reflex to offer and ask for help is gifted to us by the Earth element and it requires little or no effort when it rises from within. Nature is probably the greatest example of reciprocity. The five elements work in perfect harmony, creating and controlling each other with the innate understanding that without each other they are nothing. Each element is one constituent part of the whole. When we look at the sequential emergence of the five elements, it is the Earth element that appears last. Earth is the culmination of the life process, the manifestation of life in form, born of the other four elements. The Earth element puts the flesh on the bones of evolution, so to speak. Understanding how the cycle of life works helps us to understand our own formation. Our body, our thoughts and our feelings are all the outcome of a complex life process, brought into being by the Earth element. Like a playwright, it gathers together the disparate strands of our lives and organises them into a coherent whole with a beginning, a middle and an end. As each day draws to a close, our experience settles within us and gives us a sense of completion. George had been on this earth for a quarter of a century, yet there was no sense of satisfaction or fulfilment. His behaviour was petulant and his unwillingness to tell me why he had been referred to me was more befitting of a child than a twenty-five year-old man.

"George, help me out here. What happened?"

"Look, I kept telling her to shut up but she wouldn't,

so I decided to do something about it."

"Go on."

"I'm a member of an online group and one of the things we do is shut people down on social channels."

"You mean you were abusing her online?"

"I wouldn't call it abuse. It's standing up for what's right. We have anonymous accounts and we use them to discredit people we don't like."

"And what kind of people don't you like?"

"People with left-wing agendas. Snowflakes."

I was gobsmacked. Some of George's comments were jarring, to say the least, but I hadn't for a moment imagined that he was a cyber bully. All of a sudden I found myself reframing him in my mind as a far-right troll, which was completely at odds with my experience of him in person, when he seemed amiable, if a little difficult. It was a confusing contradiction.

"So where does Jessica come into all of this?"

"She caught me posting something."

"At work?"

He blushed. "No, I was at her place."

I thought better than to delve deeper in our first session, but his embarrassment spoke volumes, as did his unrepentant manner. He clearly believed that he hadn't done anything wrong and it was obvious that the only reason he was in my treatment room was to placate Jessica, with whom he appeared to be having more than a professional relationship.

"OK, George, let's get you on the treatment couch. Shoes and socks off, please, and your shirt, too."

I left the room to wash my hands and began reflecting on what I had learned about this enigmatic young man. My instinct was to mother him, such was his childlike demeanour, but he also had a darker side that triggered altogether different emotions within me. What was the reason for this contradiction? I wondered. Had he been influenced by someone or something in his childhood or was it something more fundamental? If I could complete my diagnosis and identify the causal element, then the answers would likely begin to reveal themselves, but so far I had only ticked two of the four boxes: odour and emotion. There was a distinct sound in his voice, but was it closer to shouting or singing? And what was the inappropriate colour I was noticing to the side of each eye? Was it the yellow we see coming from the Earth element, or a yellowy green, the distress call of the Wood element? These moments of insecurity are common for the Five-Element acupuncturist and they are important, too. If certainty comes too easily, that's precisely the moment to ask questions of oneself. Humility and the willingness to be wrong are essential. I made a note of my mental ramblings and quickly brought all of my attention back to my senses before returning to the room. As long as I was in my head, I wouldn't be able to see what Nature was showing me. George was lying on his back but had propped himself up with his elbows so he could survey the room.

"Why do you have a Buddha statue in here? Are you a Buddhist?"

"No, I just like the peaceful symbolism."

"It's cool. I wouldn't mind getting one myself. I meditate sometimes, you know?"

"That's great, George. I imagine it helps with your anxiety."

"You know, while you were washing your hands, I was thinking about the whole situation with Lucy. Maybe it was a bit mean to troll her, you know? I mean, it's not her fault she's into women and I guess she just wants to help other people who have the same problem."

"You think she has a problem?"

"Well, it's not normal, is it? Still, I gotta say she really knows her plants and when she's not being sarcastic she's actually quite interesting. She has a degree in horticulture and she used to work at the Eden Project, you know? I'd really love to get a job there."

George's voice was rich and full, yet I was struck by the constant undertone of complaint. No matter what he talked about, it was the same: the sound of someone with a problem who needs to be heard and understood. I was as sure as I could be that this was the 'sing', the sound associated with the Earth element. I couldn't confirm my diagnosis yet, as I was still unsure about his colour. Nevertheless, I felt I had enough evidence to treat him on Earth with a sufficient degree of confidence. Besides, even if my diagnosis were to change, the treatment could only be beneficial. I needled the source points of the Earth element and decided to leave it at that as the pulses had responded well and he had visibly relaxed. George clambered off the bed and dressed himself, all the while vying for my attention with a stream of questions and observations.

"One last thing, George. I get the impression that you spend a lot of time online. My job is to help you find balance and be well, so in order for this process to work it would be really helpful if you could give more of your attention to the real world rather than engaging with people online. Do you think you can manage that?"

"You want me to stay off the internet?"

"You can use your email, but given that those forums are part of the reason you're here, I suggest that you stay away from them for now."

He smiled at me. "Whatever you say. I like a good challenge." I walked over to the door and opened it for him, but when I turned round he was standing by the pot plant on my desk, gently dusting the leaves. "Succulents like a nice shiny leaf, did you know that?"

"I didn't, but it makes sense. We all want to look good, don't we?" It was a fascinating experience being with George. I was drawn to care for him but the story of his online trolling was profoundly troubling.

"Thanks, Gerad, that was fun." George had walked over to the door but seemed reluctant to leave the room.

"It was my pleasure, George. I look forward to seeing you next week. Take care." He looked at me longingly and then stepped into the corridor. I closed the door behind him, but just as I was about to sit down at my desk there was a knock and he reappeared.

"Sorry, I just want to make sure I've understood everything correctly. So, I've got to stay offline and... was there anything else? Did you want me to go for any tests?"

'You're all good, George. I'll see you next week."

EARTH MOTIVATOR

* * *

The following Tuesday, George didn't show up at the appointed time. I waited half an hour and then decided to go for a stroll in the late summer sunshine. As I opened the door to leave the building, I saw George chaining his bike to the railing on the opposite side of the street. He was covered in mud and gasping for breath.

"George! I just sent you an email. Your appointment was half an hour ago, so I assumed you weren't coming."

"I'm so sorry. I was digging out a pond and I completely lost track of time."

"Don't worry, you're in luck. My next patient is also running late." I was loath to rush a treatment but once again I found myself wanting to mother him. As soon as we walked into the treatment room, he stretched his arms slowly above his head and let out a long, loud yawn.

"You seem well, George."

"Yeah, I feel good. I'm just knackered."

He fell into the armchair, yawned a second time and started drumming his chest with both hands. His demeanour was very different from the first visit. His manner with me was open and easy and he seemed more relaxed. Too relaxed, in fact. He had slid back so far in the armchair that he was now almost horizontal and his legs were resting either side of my own. I pulled my legs back and sat upright to suggest that our session was about to begin, but George was oblivious to the cue. He had another stretch and then rested his head against the back of the chair with his eyes closed.

"George, we don't have that much time, so we need to crack on." His apparent indifference to having turned up late was striking. Was this the selfish teenager within or did he simply place no value on the help I was offering him? "So, did you manage to stay offline?"

"Hundred per cent. I read a book instead."

"Oh, anything interesting?"

"Essential. It's called 'Agenda 2030'. You should read it."

"Really? Why?"

"Basically, it explains what's really going on behind the scenes. It's terrifying. The world is controlled by a small group of people who want to impose Marxist authoritarian rule on all of us. All that wokery is just the tip of the iceberg. In the very near future we'll be living in a capitalist surveillance dystopia. Can you imagine? We haven't seen anything yet, I can tell you. The Covid lockdowns were just the beginning. We have to fight it or we're fucked."

George saw himself as a warrior fighting a sinister conspiracy, but once again his delivery made him sound more like a child complaining that he couldn't stay up late. The yellow emanating from the area around his temples had the seductive quality of a ripe peach, and he had leaned so far forward in his chair that his cloying odour had enveloped me. The appeal to join him in the centre of our shared space was palpable.

"George, I admire your passion. It's important that young people care about the future, but it seems like you're wedded to one way of thinking."

He looked furious and pressed his fists against his hips to show his indignation. "I'm wedded to the right way, that's all. My dad had good values, you know? He taught me what a proper, traditional society should look like."

My observation seemed to have rattled him. "What's up, George?"

He sank back in his chair and pouted. "Nothing." George's behaviour was fascinating but my job was to observe it, not draw psychological conclusions. My only concern was to pay attention to what the officials were asking for in order to deliver the most effective treatment. My experience in the room was of someone difficult and touchy. He desperately wanted my attention but seemed to enjoy pushing me away. This push/pull dynamic is easily understood when we look at it through the lens of the Earth element. The Earth is the central point of gravity in body, mind and spirit. It provides the foundation, stability and movement for all the other officials. The Liver official, for example, cannot make its plan without the strength and nourishment that is supplied by the Earth element, nor can the Lung official 'receive the heavenly qi' unless it is grounded by the Earth. This dependence on the Earth element is key to understanding how balance and harmony are maintained within an ever-changing cycle.

George's late arrival had cut our time together in half, so after quickly establishing what was needed, I asked him to get on the treatment couch so we could begin. It was early September now and, having checked the pulses, I decided to needle two powerful points related to the season. Every meridian has what are known as 'horary' points that emphasise the unique role and power of its officials. By stimulating these points in their respective season, all the officials benefit from an enhanced sense of stability and movement. I quickly got to work locating the first of the two points on his lower leg. As I palpated the muscle, I was struck by how dense and unyielding the flesh felt beneath my hand. The Earth element and its officials create and govern the flesh, the meat on the bone of life. The Stomach official, which governs all descending energy or 'qi', is responsible for the 'rotting and ripening' of everything we experience until it is ready for assimilation into the body, mind and spirit. The Spleen official, which governs all ascending energy, is considered to be the minister of transportation, taking the life-sustaining nourishment of our entire experience and distributing it to wherever it is needed. Everything that moves does so by the grace of the Spleen Official. When it starts to fail in its remit, there is accumulation and congestion, overthinking and worrying. Engaging with George felt like wading through mud. His words and gestures felt laboured and even when he wasn't speaking, there was a feeling of anxiety in the room.

I checked the pulses again and made a note of the readings. I was happy with the way that they had responded.

"OK, George. We're done for today."

"What? Only two points?"

"Yes, George. Your pulses feel great. That'll do."

After he left, I felt a wave of compassion for him. Part of me was irritated by his behaviour and troubled by his beliefs, yet I couldn't help feeling sorry for him. He was clearly insecure and suffering, which meant that I would need to show tolerance and understanding in order to maintain rapport. The distress call from the officials was loud and clear. They were desperate to be released from the circling morass that was the outcome of the Spleen's inability to keep everything moving.

* * *

George arrived fifteen minutes early for his third treatment. I was still with one of my other patients when I heard someone tapping on the door. I opened it to find George standing in the corridor, spinning a bunch of keys on his finger.

"Hello, Gerad! There was nobody on reception. I was worried you weren't here."

"Oh, hello, George. I'm still with a patient. Have a seat upstairs and I'll be with you shortly, OK?"

He looked dejected and turned to walk back upstairs. I was momentarily annoyed by the intrusion but, as ever, his energy and demeanour made me feel anxious and protective. As soon as I finished with my patient, I hurried upstairs to collect him, conscious of my instinct to mother him, and led him back to my treatment room.

"How are you getting on, George?"

"It's been an odd week but I feel good. I've been working flat out to get the pond in my garden finished. I've been putting it off for ages but it's coming together now. Oh, and by the way, I have a confession." He tilted his head to one side and looked at me with a doe-eyed expression. "I went online to find out where to buy goldfish." He waited for me to absolve him of his sin but I didn't react, so he pulled out his phone and showed me a picture of his soon-to-be pond. "Isn't it great? You can come and see it if you like." The picture showed a large hole in the middle of his garden, which looked more like a junkyard.

"Looks great, George. Well done. What's all the other stuff?"

"Just things I've collected over the years. I don't like to throw things away. You never know when you might need something."

One of the great attributes of the Earth element is its power to empty and keep things moving to make space for the new. Seeing the accumulation of objects in George's garden served as a metaphor for George's inner state. His blocked and compacted thinking, his hard and immovable flesh and his inability to derive satisfaction from his many blessings were vivid illustrations of the Spleen official failing to maintain the healthy movement of the cycle of life.

"You said it was an odd week. What was odd?"

"I kept thinking about my mum and it made me really sad. She suffered for years with terrible cluster headaches, you know?" He ran his weathered hands through his hair and shook his head from side to side. "Dad tried to look after her but there was nothing he could do. It turned out that she had a malignant brain tumour."

"I'm sorry to hear that, George. Can you tell me a bit more about her? About your family life? We haven't talked much about your upbringing before, have we?"

George furrowed his brow and looked at me with desperate eyes. "I'm an orphan. Did I tell you that?"

Apart from having been adopted, the childhood he described seemed perfectly normal at first, but little by little, a picture emerged of a darker world – one of gaslighting and misogyny – to which George seemed oblivious. His father idolised the Queen and Margaret Thatcher, whose portraits adorned the mantelpiece of the living room, while 'ordinary' women seemed to have been held in contempt. From what I could gather, George's mother had been treated as little more than a servant. Her role was to look after the men in her life and she, along with her desires and opinions, had been relegated to the back seat. Literally. George recalled a holiday in the Lake District when he was ten. Again, it all seemed normal, except for the fact that he sat up front with his father for the entire trip.

"Why was your mother in the back of the car?"

George looked baffled. "I don't understand the question. Isn't that normal?"

George's mother died when he was thirteen and he began to withdraw. Every evening he spent hours in online chat rooms and gradually became hooked on conspiracy theories. On weekends, he would get up early to swim in a nearby lake or go on a long-distance run. The only time he wasn't alone was when he was helping his father in the garden.

"We built a shed and a greenhouse together but my favourite thing was digging. Apparently, it started when

I was a toddler. My dad said I used to spend the whole day making holes in the sand when we went on holiday. I would shape each one into a perfect circle, fill it in and then start again."

Five years after the death of his mother, George's father was killed in a road accident. All of a sudden, he was alone in the world. An eighteen-year-old boy with a three-bedroom house in West London and enough money to ensure that he would never go hungry. Yet he had no idea how to look after himself. "My aunt came over from Canada for a few weeks but she had to go back to her own family, so she arranged for someone to cook and clean for me. Pretty soon after that I got a job with a gardening company. I didn't want to sit around doing nothing, you know? That was when I met Jessica. We were hired to work on a big landscaping project that she was designing. We hit it off, and when the job was over she asked me to go and work for her."

"How did you cope with losing your parents at such a young age?"

"It was a shock when my dad died. I really looked up to him. I was devastated."

"What about your mother?"

"Honestly, I have no idea how I coped. I remember being told that she had died but I have no recollection of how I felt. That's why it's so odd that I keep thinking about her. I'm not one for nostalgia but I've been looking at old photos and I suddenly feel quite lonely. Plus, Jessica won't see me at the moment and I miss watching movies with her."

EARTH MOTIVATOR

As Jessica was one of my patients, I was careful to avoid merging their two stories. Nevertheless, she and George were obviously in some kind of a relationship, so it was strange that she had never spoken of him as anything other than an employee. Regardless, it was encouraging to hear George open up about himself with such compassion. Something had clearly shifted in him since the second treatment. Since I was happy with the progress and confident that my diagnosis of Earth as the Causative Factor was correct, I chose two further points that would help stabilise him and provide the inner security to continue working through his personal inventory.

In the ancient Chinese tradition, the centre of the body was considered to be the umbilicus. The Stomach and Spleen meridians run in parallel on either side, holding the centre ground to govern all ascending and descending movements of qi. 'Heavenly Pivot' and 'Great Horizontal', which are two points on the Stomach and Spleen meridians respectively, lie at the same level as the umbilicus. Between them, they ensure that we never lose our central point of gravity as we negotiate the ever-changing landscape of our life.

* * *

As much as I love the dry heat of high summer, there is something rather delicious about the warm, humid air of late summer. The fluffy cumulus clouds that fill the sky herald a time of change as the Earth element begins its descent into autumn, the season of the Metal. It was now mid-September and London was enjoying an Indian summer, the consolation prize for having endured another British one. Temperatures were in the high twenties and a storm was brewing. I was standing in the reception area when a flash of lightning lit up the sky, followed by a huge thunder clap that shook the building. Two minutes later, the door opened and a rather flustered Eszter appeared, drenched from head to foot. Her normally spiky peroxide hair was hanging over her forehead like strands of spaghetti and her eyebrows had disappeared. I couldn't stop myself from laughing out loud.

"Stop it, Gerad, it's not funny. And your patient is here." She stepped aside to reveal the bedraggled figure of George, who was looking distinctly morose.

"George! You look like you've been swimming in your pond. Come on in." He barely acknowledged me and headed for the waiting room with a troubled look on his face. "You can come straight down, George, I'm ready for you." He was barely able to make eye contact, and as we made our way downstairs, I could feel a growing anxiety in the pit of my stomach. He wiped his shoes on the backs of his trouser legs and threw his coat onto the floor beneath the coat stand. "Let me hang your coat on the radiator to dry. It's soaked."

"No, leave it. It's OK."

He sat down and started wringing his hands, his head hung low. I stayed silent to see what he would do, but the atmosphere in the room intensified and he seemed to be growing increasingly agitated.

"George? What happened?"

He started pulling at his cheeks, his eyes fixed on the floor between his feet. He looked hurt and abandoned.

"I fucked up again. I blew it with Jessica."

He lifted his head and looked at me mournfully. It was a clear invitation for me to prise the information out of him, but rather than do the work for him, I waited to see if he was capable of engaging with me as an adult. We sat in silence for a while until it became clear that he wasn't going to be the one to speak.

"Would you like to tell me what happened?"

"I've just come from the police station. I've been given a warning."

"OK, can you fill me in with the whole story?"

"You know, I felt really good after our last session. I don't know if it was the needles or just talking to you about my mum. Either way, I felt great. I called Jessica and we talked for ages. I asked if I could go back to work and she said that if I sat with her and Lucy and apologised for what happened then she would be happy for me to come back." As George spoke, the tension in the room dissipated; however, it was short-lived. "Today was my first day back. I was feeling good when I arrived but the minute I saw Lucy's smug face it fucking irritated me. I tried to apologise but she started accusing me of abuse and homophobia and it just really wound me up. When Jessica stepped in and asked us to shake hands, Lucy refused and I just saw red." George rose from his chair and started pacing around the room, his feet landing heavily on the floor with each step.

"Do you want to tell me what happened after that?"

George turned to face me and brought the palms of his hands together as if in prayer. "I pushed her. I didn't think it was that hard but she fell backwards and smashed her head on the corner of the table. It was awful." He began squeezing his fists one after the other as his eyes welled up with tears. "There was blood everywhere. I didn't know what to do, so I just left. The police came round to my house that afternoon and said that Lucy had reported me. She doesn't want to press charges but they've given me a caution."

"Blimey, George. You don't make things easy for yourself, do you?"

He looked infuriated. "I'm going to leave now. I need to sort my life out." He grabbed his coat from the floor, flung open the door and stepped into the corridor, pausing briefly to look back at me. In that moment, everything about him – the look in his eyes, the furrowed brow, the slumped shoulders, the downturned mouth – all of it spoke of a desperate need to be understood.

* * *

The following week, Jessica called to apologise. I told her there was no need and asked her to tell George that if he wanted to return for treatment my door would always be open. The following day, George sent me an email, and before I knew it, he was back in my treatment room. I was pleased that he had returned because, despite the drama of the past few days, I could see that he was making progress.

"I seem to spend my whole life apologising to people."

"Is that your way of apologising to me?'

He smiled warmly and sank into the chair as if he had just arrived home.

"I felt really bad about walking out like that. I'm sorry. I couldn't handle it."

"It's OK, George. We all have our moments. So, what's your lesson from all this?"

"I've learned that I need to be more tolerant of people who aren't like me, even if I can't bear them. They have a right to be the way they are."

"That's a big lesson, George. Very Zen." George laughed and for the first time I felt as if I were engaging with an adult.

"Gerad, there's something I need to talk to you about."

"Tell me."

"Last week after the police left, I… Well, I made a bit of a shocking discovery."

"Go on."

"I was listening to a playlist on Spotify and one of the tracks triggered some really confusing emotions in me. It was a song that my mum used to play all the time. It transported me back to my childhood, and I could remember exactly how it was to be with her. The way she smelled, the sound of her voice, the way it felt to be held by her. It was such a beautiful feeling but my head was telling me to push it away. I could hear my dad's voice. It was like he was standing between me and my memories. I was scared of him, you know. I didn't dare let him know that I needed her." George pulled a tissue from his jeans and wiped away the tears that were rolling down his cheeks. "I went to her old sewing room and started leafing through the books that she used to read me when I was small. One of them had a sealed envelope in it. It was addressed to me."

The sudden twist in his story gave me goosebumps. "Who was it from?"

"Mum. It was a farewell letter. She wrote it the night before she took her life."

"I don't understand, George. You told me that she died of a brain tumour."

"I know, because that's what my dad told me. Obviously he lied to me. In the letter, mum wrote that her cluster headaches were so severe that she couldn't bear to carry on living." George's face was wracked with pain and he was fighting back the tears. "She said that my dad didn't understand, so she wanted me to know the truth. She apologised for abandoning me and asked for my forgiveness."

It's hard to convey the depth of sadness that filled the room that day. George's pain was palpable and profound. Being so close to another person's suffering is an honour but it is also a responsibility. The emotion associated with the Earth element is sympathy, which is both given and received. This emotion is a natural reflex but the extent to which we express it depends on our willingness to share another person's pain. To truly sympathise with someone involves more than offering them a shoulder to cry on; it means being willing to embody their pain, process their experience from an objective standpoint and then hand it back to them in a more digestible form. The burden of their pain is shared and then lessened, whether it is with a look, some carefully chosen words or a simple gesture of kindness. Sympathy lessens the emotional burden because the pain is genuinely shared. George's story was not my story, yet in this most intimate moment I was able to share this difficult experience.

"George, I can only imagine how hard this must be. Have you told anyone else?"

"There's no one else to tell. I have no other family."

"What about Jessica? You're close with her, no?"

"She doesn't want to see me again."

George craved attention and he had always responded positively to my gestures of care and comfort, but it was time for him to parent himself, to understand his needs and work out how to satisfy them. The first stage of this natural process was to shed the old and make space for the new. 'Abdomen Sorrow' is a point on the Spleen official's meridian and, as the name suggests, it is located in the centre of the body. In the ancient Chinese tradition, the abdomen represents the central point of our existence, the place where all of life's experiences come together, layer upon layer. But our experiences are inherently transient. Attaching to them serves only to block the natural flow of life. We are all somewhat familiar with the body's digestive process. We know that we have the capacity to ingest various forms of matter and transform them into life-sustaining energy. But this transformative process, governed by the Spleen official, also applies to thoughts, memories, emotions and ideas about ourselves. The word 'sorrow' in the name of this point refers to the inevitable loss of everything that we hold dear. Nothing in this life is permanent, so even the things that bring us the most joy are tinged with sorrow because they also contain the promise of loss.

George had experienced profound loss at a young age and the discovery of the way in which his mother had died dealt a further, agonising blow, but Nature gives us the capacity to recover from almost anything when our twelve officials are working in harmony. Central to this process of recovery is the Earth element, which enables us to endure even the most cataclysmic changes and find security and stability within. I had a strong sense that the treatment that day would be pivotal in George's transformation from hurt, abandoned child to self-sufficient adult with the ability to enter into a reciprocal relationship with life. After needling 'Abdomen Sorrow', I chose a point on the Stomach meridian called 'Receiving Fullness' that would support this moment of transformation by igniting the possibility of receiving the new.

* * *

My job is not to psychoanalyse my patients, but I felt that George wouldn't be able to fully process his past unless he had the chance to speak about it, so I made sure that I gave him enough time during our sessions to reflect on the past. It was interesting to observe his growing capacity to recall the more painful aspects of his life and either transform them into something beneficial or discard them and move on. Little by little, his outlook on life morphed from self-pity and regret to excitement and optimism. When he first came to me, his appeal for care and understanding was almost overwhelming, but now I found myself in the company of someone with whom I could have a dynamic and fun-filled interaction. After three months of twice-weekly treatments, he announced that he was going to do something that he had never before dreamed was possible. He had adopted a rescue dog called Buster, bought a small camper van and would soon be leaving to travel around mainland Europe.

I clasped George's hands in mine and congratulated him. "I feel like a proud father, you know?"

George beamed. "I really can't tell you how different I feel. When I was filling in the form to adopt Buster, I felt like a grown-up for the first time. That feeling of taking responsibility for another life is unlike anything I've ever felt. It seemed to cement everything I've been feeling recently, all of the ways I've changed."

Although moments like this give me a feeling of pride and satisfaction, I am careful not to get attached to it. In the Huangdi Neijing, the founders of this system of medicine warn against prolonged celebrations of a positive outcome, suggesting instead that the practitioner should take a brief moment to smile before moving on. In the same way, any attachment to future outcomes is inappropriate. The patient's transformation must happen – or not happen – irrespective of the practitioner's own personal desires. The Earth element plays a vital role in the patient/practitioner relationship. While we are not parents, advisors or psychotherapists, empathy is nevertheless an essential part of the healing process. Without a willingness to embody someone else's experience, it is impossible to enter into the space where healing occurs. So it is only by being an 'instrument of Nature' and drawing on the power of the Earth element that the practitioner is able to facilitate the patient's transformation without forming personal attachments that may get in the way.

A year later, I was leaving the clinic one evening when someone came screeching to a halt on a bicycle. It was George, and he was grinning from ear to ear. With breathless excitement, he told me about his adventures in Spain and Portugal, how he had walked in the Pyrenees and run with the bulls in Pamplona, how he and Buster had dug holes in the sand together and, most importantly of all, how he had met a girl called Carla in Lisbon.

"She's three months pregnant, Gerad. I'm going to be a dad!" As the stories poured out of him I couldn't help but marvel at the sight of the confident, grounded young man in front of me. He still wanted my attention and approval, but it seemed much more natural. The desperation was gone and I was only too happy to be part of such a joyful and reciprocal encounter.

7
FLY AND SCATTER

*

Alice was hanging her coat on the back of the door when she suddenly jumped.

"What was that?"

"What was what?"

"That rumbling noise. It sounded like horses running."

"Oh, that's the tube. The trains pass right underneath the building. I'm surprised you haven't noticed it before." I had been seeing Alice for about ten years but her visits were sporadic at best, so her file had been relegated to the section of my filing cabinet reserved for 'boom and bust' patients. Typically, this group of patients contact me once in a blue moon asking for an urgent appointment, attend three to five sessions and then disappear until the next crisis comes along. I retrieved her file from the vault, sat down opposite her and began reading the notes from our last session.

"It's been two years, Alice. I'm happy to see you again." Alice had perched on the edge of her chair, her hands clasping the seat cushion. She looked at me nervously before breaking into a smile and sighing.

"I'm happy to see you, too, Gerad. You're always here, thank God. You always look the same. It's so reassuring. It's like time and everything that happens in between my visits evaporates within seconds of entering the room."

Alice was a tall, intense woman in her mid-thirties with short dark hair, high cheekbones and dark brown eyes. She only ever dressed in black, offset by ruby-red lipstick and the occasional sliver of white from a handkerchief stuffed artfully into the breast pocket of her suit jacket. Her facial features were androgynous, yet years of dancing had given her a fluidity of movement that was distinctly feminine. She had originally come to me when she was twenty-five, suffering from headaches, chronically dry skin and shin splints. At the time she was working as a dancer and choreographer and had formed her own company to explore what she called "lesbians' uneasy relationship to the cis-hetero form of ballet". I had no idea what that meant but I was wary of asking, so I scribbled it down word for word in case I ever needed to talk about her work in the future. She also told me that she identified as non-binary and liked to be addressed as she/her. When she asked me how I liked to be addressed, I panicked and said "me/mine", which thankfully she found amusing. Ten years on, her life looked very different. She was still a dancer, but for the past few years she had been living as part of a 'throuple' with an older woman and a younger man in a large house in North London. Their rather unconventional household was completed by two dogs, three cats and a large snake called Hydra.

FLY AND SCATTER

"How are you, Alice?"

"My goodness, where do I start?" She looked at me quizzically as if she were expecting me to answer her question, but just as I was about to speak she held her head in her hands and let out a scream. "Arghhh! They're so fucking annoying." I was taken aback by her outburst but I tried not to let it show and continued with my line of questioning, speaking calmly and quietly.

"Who's annoying, Alice?" Rather than steady her, this innocent question burst the dam and she launched into an hysterical rant, which gushed out with a force of emotion that I found quite unsettling. It appeared that her partners, Alexandra and Christian, were constantly at each other's throats, yet somehow she was always to blame. Then there was the money. Alice was the only breadwinner in the household, but they never showed any kind of gratitude.

"And that's not all. My agent has arranged an audition for me in Los Angeles and it's everything I've ever dreamed of and Alexandra and Christian are urging me to go but they know I can't because of my fear of flying and they just think I'm being weak and..." I remained quiet and waited for her to settle down again. "What do you think, Gerad? I need to do this. It's a once-in-a-lifetime opportunity and I would do anything to escape, but how? There's no way I can fly unless they knock me out with an elephant tranquilliser and stick me in the hold." I wanted to laugh, but she wasn't trying to be funny. On the contrary, she was clearly in a state of panic and despair.

"Alice, I think we need to put all of this in the right

context. Is the trouble at home because you are stressed about the casting, or is it your fear of flying? Or is it something else, perhaps?"

Her eyes began to fill with tears. "I... don't... know... Everything?" All of a sudden, she looked like a lost child, consumed by fear. I leaned forward and took her hands but it was too late. The flood gates had opened and it was a full two minutes before the shaking, spluttering and weeping finally came to a halt, at which point she straightened her back and popped her knuckles. This pattern was familiar to both of us. Alice would arrive, take a short while to settle and then a tsunami would erupt from her depths, overwhelm the room and pass.

"Better?"

"Much better, thank you."

"What's the casting for, Alice?"

"It's for the lead role in a movie. It's the story of a young woman who pretends to be a man and becomes the principal dancer at the State Opera."

"That's quite a story, Alice. You're perfect for it. Let's get you out of here and on that plane to Los Angeles." The horses charged through the room again but this time she was oblivious to the noise. Her attention seemed to have gone elsewhere.

* * *

Alice's first visit to me ten years earlier had been nothing short of extraordinary. I had scheduled my normal ninety minutes for the initial consultation, but I quickly realised this wouldn't be long enough unless I could stem the flow of stories and emotions. Early on in the session, she dropped the first of many bombshells.

"My mother hated me from the moment I was born. She thought there was something wrong with me because I refused to breastfeed and screamed whenever she picked me up. Apparently I never smiled."

"Who told you this? I assume you don't remember?"

"My aunt told me. When I was ten, Mummy was sectioned, so Auntie had to step in and look after me. Somewhere inside I must have known that there was something wrong with her, even as a small child. My earliest memories are of being dressed in little outfits that Mummy had the housekeeper make for me. They were identical to her own. She would make me stand next to her in front of the mirror and proudly tell me that we were the same person." Alice smiled but her icy stare betrayed an altogether darker emotion. "She was mad as a hatter but I didn't know anything different, so to me it all seemed quite normal at the time. It was only in retrospect that I could see how crazy it all was. And it wasn't until I was in my twenties that I understood why."

"What do you mean by that?"

"Her own mother was even crazier than she was. When Mummy was two years old, Granny upped sticks and travelled to Cairo, where she partied until the end of the war. She had the housekeeper sew swastikas into her underwear in case she was caught by the Germans en route. When she came back after the war, my mother didn't know who she was."

"That's quite a story, Alice. Where were you living when your mother was sectioned?"

"I lived with Auntie at the London house and then when I was eleven we moved back to the estate in Scotland where I was home-schooled. I hated it. It was damp and dreary."

"That sounds so disturbing and scary for a girl of your age. How did you feel being away from everything you knew?"

"I was miserable. I remember sitting on a large window ledge, the cold stone burning into my legs, staring out at the bleak landscape. It was awful. I can still remember the nagging feeling of dread. It lives inside me."

"Where was your father?"

"He was there but I hardly ever saw him. He was busy with the estate. When I was thirteen, I was sent away to boarding school. It was clear that Mummy wasn't going to be coming home and there was a problem with Rory." The casual way in which Alice threw this "problem" into the conversation made it sound unimportant, an incidental detail that she had almost forgotten to mention, but I sensed that there was more to it than that.

"Who was Rory?"

"The estate manager. He was an older man, very good-looking with dark, wavy hair. I really liked him but when my father was away he would get drunk and do weird things." She stared at me vacantly for a moment. "I had a pony called Bonnie and I was grooming her in the stables one day when Rory came in and bolted the door. He was completely out of it. He picked me up and placed me on top of the hay bales. He said that if I tried to get away he would tell my father what we were doing together."

"Did he hurt you?"

"Not me, no. It was Bonnie he hurt. He violated her in front of me. It happened on and off for about two years. At first he just made me watch but one day he started trying to touch me. I managed to get away but the next day my father called me into his study and told me that he was sending me away to boarding school."

"Did he give you a reason?"

"He just said he thought it was for the best."

"I'm so sorry you had to go through all these horrendous experiences, Alice. Did you speak to anyone about the abuse?"

"Abuse? It's normal. Everyone has weird shit going on in their childhood." I have heard a lot of disturbing stories over the years, but these deeply troubling disclosures and the way Alice described them shocked me to the core. I looked into her staring eyes to see if I could get a sense of what she was feeling. There was no way through. She seemed to be emotionally petrified.

When Alice first came to see me, I remember thinking that if anyone wanted evidence of the Causative Factor and the way that it is diagnosed through colour, sound, odour and emotion, they need only meet Alice to be convinced. When I called out her name in the waiting room, I remember the intense feeling of drama as this tall, statuesque figure rose from her chair, straightened her jacket and locked eyes with me. I immediately felt on edge. "Where are we going?" she asked as I led the way down to my treatment room. She seemed suspicious and kept looking over her shoulder as if she were charting the way out should the need suddenly arise. When someone gives off such an obvious and inappropriate sense of unease, I automatically wonder if it is one of the distress calls of the Water element and its associated emotion, fear. It was too soon to say if this was the case, but the odour that emanated from her as she walked past me to enter the treatment room suggested that it might be. Every cell in our body is made up of about seventy per cent water, which is recycled by a process of osmosis. When the system breaks down, the water stagnates, releasing an odour reminiscent of a damp basement.

Throughout the consultation, I felt an undercurrent of fear. Alice was restless, wary and on edge. One minute she would cup her hands and whisper something banal as if it were a carefully guarded secret, then she would ramp up the volume and rush to tell me every detail of something sensitive in a monotonous drone that would go on and on until she suddenly ran out of steam in mid-sentence. At other times she was quiet, barely responding to my questions and visibly troubled by the silence that enveloped the room. She would pick up her phone repeatedly to check that it was switched off or turn to look at the door as if she needed to remind herself where the exit was. I remember noticing the strange, murky colour around her temples. For a while I couldn't give it a label, probably because I was impatient to find the final piece of the diagnostic puzzle, but just as I was about to give up, a browny blue came into focus like the hidden picture in a three-dimensional stereogram. Once I had seen it, it was hard to believe that I hadn't noticed it before. My diagnosis was complete. I was as sure as I could be that Alice had a Causative Factor in the Water element, and it was the Kidney and Bladder officials that were disturbing the peace.

* * *

One of Alice's complaints was aerophobia. Ever since she was a child, she had been frightened of heights, but while tall buildings and bridges made her nervous, the mere mention of flying sent her into a state of wide-eyed panic. She had only ever travelled twice on a plane and on both occasions it had been a disaster. The first time was in her early twenties, when she flew to Marrakech for a modelling job. Shortly after take-off, she locked herself in the toilet and refused to come out, despite repeated appeals from the cabin crew. She took the long way home and swore never to fly again. The second attempt was a flight to New York for an audition at the Metropolitan Opera. She had paid a hefty fee to a hypnotherapist, who claimed to be able to cure her phobia in a single session, but she was so scared that she got drunk on the plane and was escorted off by the police on arrival.

Her domestic set-up was equally complicated. She had met her partner when she was an eighteen-year-old student at the Royal Ballet School in London. Alexandra was a visiting teacher from Boston and twenty-five years her senior. She was also married. Their relationship blossomed, and by the time Alice graduated from ballet school, Alexandra had left her husband and moved to London. She bought a townhouse in Shoreditch and gradually insinuated Alice into her home and her life. Alice's dancing career took off quickly and her unusual looks also caught the attention of casting directors. She was soon deriving a sizable income from modelling and acting, both of which came easily to her. Then, seven years after meeting Alexandra, Alice casually announced that the couple had become a throuple.

"He's called Christian. Alexandra met him at an awards ceremony while I was at home with the flu. Love at first sight or so they keep telling me. She brought him home that night and he's been with us ever since."

"That was quick! I know Alexandra was married to a man before but I assumed you guys were a monogamous couple."

"Labels don't interest me, Gerad. So, how are you going to cure my fear of flying?" Alice's attempt to change the subject was jarring. I had no idea how the dynamics of a *ménage à trois* played out, but something didn't feel right.

"Are you and Alexandra on the same page with this? Your new partner, I mean."

"Look, it's different for her. She's already done the whole husband and wife thing, so it's more familiar to her, but I want her to be happy and it means that when I go away to Los Angeles she'll have company." Although I wasn't convinced that Alice was telling me everything, I felt that I had no choice but to let the matter drop. Then, about a year into their new relationship, she arrived at the clinic with a brown manila folder. "Things are a bit fraught at home, so I've created a document to lay down the ground rules. It's Alexandra's house but she doesn't work any more and neither does Christian, so it's me that pays all the bills and it's doing my head in. What do you think?" She opened the folder and handed me a chunky document held together by a butterfly clip.

Alice, Alexandra and Christian
Terms & Conditions
Page 1	Housekeeping Matters
Page 5	Legal Matters
Page 8	Boundaries
Page 12	Honesty and Communication
Page 13	Pre-Throuple Life
Page 15	Resolution of Issues
Page 21	Transparency
Page 22	Finances (Group and Individual)

"That's a lot of information, Alice. Well done for creating it but I'm no expert on this kind of thing. I see there are sections on finance and legal matters, so I suggest you get someone qualified to look at it." I handed the document back to her and she promptly threw it onto the floor beside her chair. She was clearly irritated. "Alice, I hope you don't mind me asking, but are you really OK with how you're living as a throuple?"

"I'm fine. Teething problems, that's all." I already knew from our sessions together that being in control of every area of her life was very important to her. My personal experience of her in the room, which is all I have to go on when it comes to making a diagnosis, was that she was either confident and in control, panicky and out of control, or aggressive. When she was in control mode, it often felt overbearing and intrusive. She would attempt to command my space, telling me how the session should unfold in order to deliver the outcome that she wanted. Conversely, the out-of-control Alice would present as a terrified child in need of safety and reassurance. I liked her very much within the professional setting but I never knew which version of her was going to walk through the door, and it was not hard to imagine how difficult she might be to live with.

In the human body, the Water element is represented by the kidneys and the bladder. In the ancient Chinese context, the Kidney official is the "controller of the waterways" but it is the Bladder official that is given the complex task of managing the storage of water in the body, mind and spirit. Given that water is the origin of all life and makes up almost seventy per cent of our body, this is an extraordinarily important role. The Bladder official is also considered to be responsible for the cultivation of yin, the very substance of our existence. According to yin/yang theory, our world is made up of perfectly balanced and inextricably linked opposites: night and day, hot and cold, male and female, yin and yang. The evolution of the universe is entirely dependent on the subtle balance of the attracting and opposing forces that appeared at the moment of separation from the source of all creation. The yin/yang dynamic is the basis of cell division, the process of breathing and the beating of the heart. The yin aspect is one side of this dependent relationship, and it is the Bladder official that is responsible for making sure that there is enough water. Without yin, there is no yang. Without water, there is no life.

The Bladder official has the longest meridian of all the officials, with a total of sixty-seven acupuncture points starting at the inner canthus of the eyes, traversing over the head, neck, back and legs and ending up at the little toe. The final point is called 'Extremity of Yin', marking the culmination of the task of protecting and maintaining the basis of life. When the Water element and its officials are functioning as Nature ordained, they give us buoyancy and we are able to keep our head above water, so to speak. When they are not, we feel as though we are at risk of drowning, and the response is a continuous state of fear and vigilance.

'The Law of Least Action', one of the five natural laws that inform the practice of Five-Element Acupuncture, teaches us that the simplest treatments are the most powerful. I was happy with my original diagnosis, but a considerable amount of time had elapsed since I last treated Alice, and there had been some significant changes in her life, so I decided to start from the beginning. I needled the source points of the Bladder and Kidney officials to see how the other four elements and their officials would respond. My hope was that it would act as a reset and help her to get a fresh perspective on everything.

* * *

When Alice returned the following week, I was running late. She was not pleased. She pushed open the door, threw her coat on the floor and stared at me.

"I'm so sorry to keep you waiting, Alice."

"I've only got forty-five minutes so can we please just get on with it." I began asking a few questions to establish whether or not the last treatment had been effective, but she was not interested in cooperating. "These questions are not helpful. Can we just get on with the treatment?" Without waiting for an answer, she removed her shoes, got up from the chair and lay down on the treatment couch. I walked over to my desk and took a moment to compose myself.

"Alice, I think it's important for you to realise that our interaction before the treatment is not for you, it's for me. I need time to confirm my diagnosis and construct the best possible treatment." I stood by her side and took her left hand to read the pulses. "Please bear that in mind in the future." Rather than respond she tensed up even more, her eyes fixed on the ceiling. The Huangdi Neijing states that "reestablishing the balance always depends on the spirit... Without the cooperation of the patient, you cannot do your work". I needed to re-establish rapport but also reassert my authority as the 'instrument', so that I could be in direct contact with the officials through the conduit of the needles. As I moved around the couch taking her pulses, I noticed that she was fighting back tears.

"Thank you for sticking with me, Gerad." I finished the treatment and sat next to her to see how she was responding. As she lay there, her body slowly began to soften and she opened her eyes.

"Have you been to the Torture Garden, Gerad?"

"No, but I've heard of it. It's a fetish club, right?"

"Yes. Alexandra and Christian have started taking me there." She sat up, swung her legs over the treatment couch and began regaling me with stories of the weird and wonderful world of the club. "There's an area called The Playroom at the end of a long corridor with red padded walls. It has every kind of sex toy you can imagine. Everyone does whatever they want in there."

"Do *you* enjoy The Playroom, Alice?"

"Alexandra is the queen of the room and Christian is her servant."

"What about you, Alice? What's your role?"

"I just watch them."

* * *

For most of my younger years, winter felt like something I had to endure. I yearned for long, hot, sunny days and the freedom to spend time outside. When I started my training in acupuncture, however, I began to see the beauty and importance of each and every season, including my old foe. After the excitement and abundance of summer, winter invites us to retreat, rest and look within. This process of introspection and what it reveals, both positive and negative, builds and strengthens us so that when the spring comes, we are able to burst forth with renewed energy and vigour. But what Chinese medicine also teaches us is that we can draw on these seasonal qualities at any time. The capacity to rest safely and peacefully, to stay calm in the face of chaos or danger, to find our inner drive and power to fulfil our dreams; all of these wonderful attributes that we observe in Nature are there for us when the Water element is functioning as it should. On a crisp, cold morning in December, I arrived at the clinic to find Eszter attaching baubles to the fake Christmas tree that was about to take up its annual residence in front of the fireplace in our reception area.

"Can't we get a new tree, Eszter? It's so ugly." Eszter raised a finger to her lips and pointed to the waiting room. I popped my head round the corner and saw a familiar figure standing by the window with her back to me, dressed from head to toe in black. Despite my assertion of authority in our previous session, the sight of Alice still triggered a feeling of unease in me. She seemed to be calmer than the previous week, so I decided to steer clear of her domestic troubles, but it didn't take long before even the most innocuous questions began to ruffle her feathers. It was increasingly clear that something was getting in the way of our rapport. Historically, Alice and I had always worked well together and, even when she was facing challenges, she would be eager to tell me how much the treatments had helped her, but something had changed. This was the third treatment since she had come back to see me, yet I felt that we were further away from the desired outcome than when we first started. I was becoming increasingly concerned about her state of mind, but rather than probe further into the drama of her life and disappear down a rabbit hole, I decided to stay focused on my diagnosis and use what I was experiencing in the room to guide my treatment plan. What was going on? What were the officials asking for? As always, it was my senses that would provide the answers.

The atmosphere in the room was unsettling. The sound in her voice seemed more disturbing than ever, a monotonous rumbling that masked what she was actually saying, and her odour was more intense than ever. Before it had been like the smell of damp. Now it was more like ammonia. Her inner world was clearly in chaos and the officials were struggling to cope. But it was not just her inner world. Alice's determination to get to Los Angeles had become almost obsessive. She would frame it as a need to run towards something, the allure of Hollywood, the excitement of starring in a film, but I had a strong sense that it was the opposite, a growing and desperate need to escape. But from what? So much of Alice seemed to be hidden beneath layers of self-delusion and terror. Did she really accept her painful childhood? Was she truly approaching her relationships with a healthy, confident and self-assured mindset? It seemed to me that part of her struggle was an inability to emerge from the dark, scary place to which she must surely have retreated in order to survive her childhood. Was her current domestic situation condemning her to stay there? Only Alice would know the answers to those questions. My role was to deliver the treatments that would give her the strength and clarity she needed to seek them out.

'Eyes Bright' is the first point on the Bladder meridian,

located by the side of the nose and just into the inner canthus of the eye. This point gives us the ability to step into the light and face each new day without fear, knowing that we have everything we need to survive. It is akin to the feeling that we have after a night of deep, restorative sleep. As I positioned myself to place the needle on the skin, I noticed that she had applied heavy make-up above her right eye to cover a bruise. I inserted the needle until I felt the slight pull that told me it had reached the depth of the point. Alice sighed and relaxed. The tension in the room had dissipated but I still felt uneasy about what I had just discovered. I paused for a moment to get a sense of which point would best support the one I had just treated. 'Fly and Scatter', another point on the Bladder meridian, is located on the back of the calf muscle. Its name derives from the sight of flying insects emerging from the dark waters of winter, heralding the arrival of spring and the renewal of the life cycle. The Bladder official, responsible for maintaining our water reservoirs, must also facilitate the release of the energy that naturally accumulates within them. 'Fly and Scatter' triggers this release, alleviating stagnation, promoting flow and reinvigorating all of the officials just as the rising tide lifts all of the ships. I asked Alice to bend her legs so I could mark the point on her calf, but as I did so I noticed another bruise on her shin.

"That's quite a bruise, Alice. How did that happen?" She pulled the blanket over her legs and looked away. I stopped what I was doing, sat on the stool next to her and gently rested my hand on her forearm. "Before I carry on, Alice, I just wanted to ask if there is anything you would like to tell me. The more I know, the better equipped I am to help you."

She started to shake and tears began streaming down her cheeks.

"I'm OK, Gerad. I'm just tired. Very, very tired."

* * *

Taking full responsibility for how our life unfolds is a concept many of us shy away from. As children, we are subject to the whims of the people in whose care we find ourselves, but once we become adults, our destiny is in our own hands, in theory at least. Whether it's a hangover from childhood or part of an imbalance in one of the elements, it's often easier to see ourselves as victims than recognise that we are the architects of our own lives. When our starting point is fear and paranoia, this is especially true. The adrenalised response to routine challenges can feel like a life-or-death battle, leaving no room for the more rational voice that might step in and ask, "Hey, hang on a minute, what's really going on here?" I had never met Alexandra or Christian and I was loath to jump to conclusions based on Alice's testimony alone, but my fear was that there was something sinister going on. Her home life seemed to be one big drama after another, and the discovery of the bruises only served to exacerbate my concerns. Was this a case of domestic violence? Was this a medical red flag that I had a responsibility to pursue? Was it any of my business? I decided that I would express my concerns during the next session if it still felt appropriate, but I couldn't get her off my mind for the rest of the week.

On the morning of her next appointment, I was in the clinic bright and early. Alice always arrived for her sessions bang on time but by eight twenty there was still no sign of her. I checked my email to see if she had sent me a message but there was nothing. Eight thirty came and went. When I called her mobile, it went straight to voicemail, so I rushed upstairs to the reception area to see if Eszter had heard from her.

"What's wrong with you, Gerad? You're so jumpy. I've never seen you like this."

"I just want to get on with the day. Alice is going to throw out my whole schedule."

"She's not coming."

"What do you mean? Did she just call?"

"Last week she got into a heated argument with someone. She locked herself in the toilet and started yelling down the phone. I had to knock on the door and ask her to keep it down."

"But how do you know she's not coming today?"

"Just a feeling." Eszter's role as receptionist was deceptively simple. Far from being a paper pusher, she used her unique vantage point to study the cast of characters that passed through the clinic. She had an uncanny ability to suss people out and, in moments like this, I trusted her intuition. I went back to my room and checked the time. Alice was forty-five minutes late. I was suddenly gripped by fear as I remembered our recent conversations and the bruises on her body. What could I do? I called a colleague in confidence to ask for advice.

"Calm down, Gerad. You're not being rational. She's probably just forgotten."

"Calm down? You don't understand, she's been so anxious recently. And the bruises… I know she wasn't telling me everything." I could hear the panic in my voice as the adrenaline coursed through my veins. Maybe my colleague was right. Maybe I wasn't being rational, but the fear was in charge now. I pulled out her file, scribbled down her address and ran upstairs. "Eszter, I've got to run out. Tell my next patient there's been an emergency. I'll call you in about thirty minutes, OK?" I flagged down a taxi and asked the driver to get me there as quickly as possible, but it seemed that every red light in London was conspiring against me. I kept trying Alice's number but still it went to voicemail. Twenty minutes later, we finally pulled up outside Alice's home, a large red-brick Georgian townhouse with black shutters and spiked railings. I stepped out of the cab and took a deep breath before approaching the front door. I stood for a moment staring at the brass knocker, above which was a large Christmas wreath and a sprig of holly. I could feel my heart beating against my rib cage. I knocked and waited but there was no response, so I knocked again. Nothing. I looked up to see if there were any lights on in the house and then peered through the letterbox – still no sign of life. I turned to walk away but just as I reached the gate, I heard the rattle of a chain. The door opened and a sleepy face with deep-set wrinkles looked out at me from behind the security chain.

"Who is it?"

"Forgive me for disturbing you. You must be Alexandra. I'm Gerad, Alice's acupuncturist. Is she here?"

"Gerad? Gerad! Dear, oh dear. I'm so sorry." My heart sank. The woman unfastened the chain and opened the door. She looked weary and distressed. Come on in, Gerad. I'm on the phone but take a seat and I'll be with you in a minute." I walked into the living room and sat on the edge of one of the armchairs by an open fire, which was still glowing through a bed of ashes. On the floor beside the fireplace was an empty bottle of wine and two glasses, one of which had been knocked onto its side, leaving a deep red stain on the flagstone. On the wall above was a large painting of a young ballerina leaping into the air with her arms held aloft.

"It's a lovely painting, isn't it? Do you recognise her?" I turned around to find a tall, bearded man standing in the doorway. "I'm Christian. Good to meet you. I've heard a lot about you from Alice."

"Where is she? Is she OK? She was supposed to see me this morning."

"I know. I was supposed to call you but it's all been a bit hectic. We've been up since four this morning. I took her to the airport to catch a flight to Los Angeles. I was going to message you as soon as I got back but it completely slipped my mind. Forgive me."

I was relieved, angry and confused all at once. "She's flying to LA?"

"She sure is. Hollywood bound, my friend."

"She wasn't nervous to fly?"

"Apparently not. Alexandra pumped her full of red

wine and Valium to make absolutely sure that she wouldn't panic but she was adamant that you had cured her. Whatever it takes, right?"

* * *

When I got back to the clinic, I sent Alice an email to wish her well with the audition but she never replied. That evening, I spent some time reflecting on everything that had happened. I needed to take responsibility for my personal drama in this scenario, for somehow having got caught up in her story. Without realising it, I had built a case and drawn conclusions that were entirely rooted in my own fear response. All of it was based on the assumption that Alice's version of events was true. Maybe it was, but from personal and professional experience, I know that most of us are unreliable witnesses to the events that unfold in our own lives. We become wedded to our story, convinced that the way we see the world is the way it really is, and then we design our lives from this foundation of 'truth'. Learning about the Water element taught me that fear rises within us like the water in a reservoir, slowly growing in strength until it reaches a tipping point. When the dam bursts there is no stopping the water, and so it is with fear. I had been aware of a mounting tension within me during my sessions with Alice, but I never imagined that I would be so overwhelmed by irrational fear that I would strike out on a mission to save her.

One of the most challenging aspects of my profession is being able to listen to the never-ending dramas without getting personally involved. A patient's story can be informative, but it is of no consequence when it comes to diagnosis. The only way to know where to place the needles is to pay attention to the sensory experience of being with someone. Most of the time I am able to maintain this separation, but every once in a while, I feel myself being sucked into the story. When I was with Alice, not only did I feel the fear in the room, I also got caught up in the drama, and eventually I was swept away in a flood of fear and panic.

Every now and again, I searched online for anything that would give me the comfort of knowing that she was alive and well, but I found nothing. Occasionally, when looking for notes on one of my patients, I would come across Alice's file, and each time I had the same uneasy feeling in the pit of my stomach. It made me think of the families of missing persons for whom that sickening feeling is a daily reality, but it also reminded me of so many of my patients who carry this feeling throughout their lives, despite never having suffered any kind of trauma. For them, it is a feeling that has no apparent cause, an elemental imbalance that permeates their experience. The Water element is our silent backstory. It is our cause, our potential and the source of the reassuring sense that we can survive in this world. My experience with Alice had deepened my understanding of how, when it is in balance, this element gives us the power and drive we need to navigate the challenges of this mysterious life. Without it, we feel as though we are lost at sea.

8

PALACE OF WEARINESS

*

"Hey, hey, heyyy!" Jessie's voice was unmistakable. Joyous, upbeat and inappropriately loud. I got up from my chair to greet her, but before I could even make it to the door, a small brown and white terrier darted into the room with his tail wagging. Trailing in his wake was an extendable lead with a plastic handle, which got caught under the door, stopping him in his tracks and flipping him upside down like a beached turtle. I bent down and removed the lead, whereupon he calmly trotted over to my desk and relieved himself on the carpet. Toto belonged to Jessie and he always arrived about thirty seconds before her to prepare the ground for the drama that was about to unfold. Sure enough, just as he turned his head to inspect his handiwork, the door swung open and his owner swept into the room like a whirlwind, talking loudly into her phone.

"Jessie! Keep your voice down, please!" I shook my fists in a theatrical manner and pointed towards Toto, who was kicking up imaginary dust with his hind legs to cover up his misdemeanour. Jessie collapsed into the armchair without removing her coat and carried on talking to the person on the other end of the phone.

"Laila, gotta go. I'm with Gerad and Toto just disgraced himself. Gerad, Laila says 'hi'. I'll call you back in about an hour, OK? Toto! Stop that!" Toto was now trying to dig a hole in the corner of the room where the moths had been hard at work.

"Jessie, can we all calm down for a moment?" I grabbed the little terrier by the collar and made him sit by my chair.

Jessie was a strikingly beautiful woman in her thirties who, despite her looks, always managed to give the impression that she had just crawled out of bed. Her hair was in a permanent state of disarray, a confusion of curls that was forever getting snagged in the zip of her trademark outfit, a baggy tracksuit and a pair of fluffy suede boots that had been partially destroyed by Toto when he was a puppy. She was the definition of gregariousness, spreading herself across a vast landscape of relationships, yet she was unable to maintain a steady, open connection with anyone for more than a short while. Bite-sized phone conversations and fleeting visits were as much as she could manage, but it was these brief, intimate connections that fed her, so she poured every ounce of her energy into keeping them all alive. Then, exhausted by it all, she would retreat to her bedroom and cuddle up with Toto, while the flame that had burned so brightly would gradually flicker and die.

She had originally come to me six months earlier,

worried that what her doctor had described as "catastrophic periods" might affect her fertility. She had her sights set on a house and a family while she was still in the prime of her life, and she didn't want anything to stand in her way. Right from the start, it was clear that she was unaware of professional boundaries or generally accepted rules of conduct. She was a force of Nature – boisterous, irreverent and very funny – and I always looked forward to her visits, despite the fact that she thought it was perfectly normal to make and receive phone calls throughout the session. She would jump from one to the next without drawing breath, punctuating her conversations with shrieking laughs that drew complaints from the room next door.

"Can we skip the talking bit today?" Jessie had wrapped up the call and placed her phone face up on the arm of the chair, ready for the next one. "There's nothing to say. The periods are beyond terrible, my skin's a disaster and I've got zero energy."

"Has anything changed in your..." Before I could finish my sentence, her phone started ringing.

"Oh hello, thanks for calling me back. I wanted to book a facial... Yes, today, please... Three thirty is perfect... No, I just need you to get rid of the beard." Jessie behaved like a naughty adolescent, but she always managed to spin any misdemeanour into something charming, flirtatious and utterly delightful. When I first met her, I, like everyone else, couldn't help but fall for her. I loved her unfiltered honesty, her inappropriate behaviour and her outrageous sense of humour, but I was also drawn to her thinly veiled vulnerability, the pain in her heart that she carried so gracefully and her impulse to care for her friends. Jessie was one of those people that everyone loved to be around. There was something about her that made you feel you could tell her anything, and her warmth and generosity were seemingly boundless. She was everyone's cheerleader. Everyone's except for her own, that is.

"Jessie, we need to talk about your periods, if nothing else. If you want to get pregnant, it's essential to have a healthy menstrual cycle."

"A healthy boyfriend wouldn't go amiss either."

"I'm sorry?"

"He's driving me nuts!"

"Who? Chris?"

"Yes, Chris! I love him but sometimes I just want to strangle him. He can't even commit to looking at properties with me, let alone starting a family." Jessie generally managed to cover up the way she was feeling with banter and jokes, but for once I sensed a real frustration and sadness.

"What's holding him back?"

"I don't know, but every time I mention it he finds a way to change the subject." Her phone rang again and she plunged headlong into another conversation, seemingly oblivious to my presence or any sense of decorum. "Are you kidding? Why would I go bikini shopping with three size zero women? I'd rather go home for dinner... and not eat."

Jessie's self-deprecating humour gave her a certain kind of freedom and social currency, but behind the jokes lay a vulnerable woman who I feared might never recover. She had grown up in North London, the youngest child of wealthy textile merchants. When she was twenty-five, she fell madly in love with a man called Chris, the son of a well-known musician. He was ten years older than her and worked as an agent in the music business. Jessie was working as a producer for one of London's independent radio stations and was rapidly working her way up the ladder. A year after they met, they found a flat to rent in Soho and moved in together. Her parents were horrified. Jessie had been brought up in a very conservative family and her parents were forever preaching the importance of traditional values. Living in sin with a renowned hellraiser who shared none of their cultural or religious heritage was not what they wanted for their daughter, but the more they tried to suppress her, the more determined she was to break free. She and Chris were young, beautiful and successful. Everyone wanted to know them and they were regulars on London's party circuit. In the space of a couple of years, the kid from Stanmore had been transformed into a confident, gregarious young woman who was mixing with London's glitterati. Despite her parents' objections and constant warnings from friends, who were concerned about the debauchery of her social set, the relationship flourished and they began putting aside money to buy a property of their own.

Jessie wrapped up the call and finally turned her full attention to me. "What were we saying?"

"You were saying that you can't get Chris to look at properties with you."

"Oh, yes. Well, I guess I just have to accept the way he is, but it's so frustrating. It's hard enough trying to get my parents to accept him as part of the family, let alone convince them he's got my best interests at heart." Jessie forced a smile as she wiped away a tear.

"OK, Jessie. Let's see what we can do with the needles."

"Are you going to do the weight loss point today?"

"You know there's no such thing."

"Of course there is! You did it last time and I lost half a stone." She leapt to her feet, stripped off her top and did a spinal twist so she could see the full spectrum of her waist. "I'm off to Greece in a fortnight and I do *not* want to look like I've just been booted out of the fat farm."

"Well, there's no time to waste then. Shoes, socks and top off, please. I'll be back in a second once I've washed my hands." When I walked back into the room, Jessie was lying on the treatment couch, wriggling like a worm. She still had her boots on and Toto was curled up on the blanket at the foot of the couch, which was now covered in mud. She lifted her arms one after the other to examine her armpits and then lowered her tracksuit bottoms so she could pinch the flesh around her waist. I leaned against my desk for a moment to survey the spectacle.

"What are you waiting for, Gerad? This fat isn't going to disappear on its own."

"I'm waiting for you to remove your boots."

* * *

The standout clue to Jessie's Five-Element diagnosis was

her odour. It was the smell of something burning and, even for the untrained nose, it was impossible to miss. Sometimes it was like the steam from a tumble dryer, on other days it was like stale cigarette ash. When she was not in performance mode, her voice sounded flat and lifeless, broken only by the occasional giggle. The colour beside her eyes was ashen grey and, despite her exuberant persona, I sensed a profound lack of joy that seemed to speak of an inner pain. Jessie's Causative Factor was in the Fire Element and it was the Circulation-Sex official that was struggling to provide a consistent flow of love, warmth and openness for all the other officials.

The joyless state experienced by someone whose Fire officials are not functioning correctly is not the outcome of external circumstances. Rather, it is a symptom of the Fire struggling to find the heat, fuel and oxygen that it needs to produce the feeling of light and warmth within. When this ashen state becomes the dominant paradigm of a person's being, they have two choices: retreat to the lonely but safe harbour within, or reach out to the world in search of the warmth and love that other people provide. On the surface, such outward gestures of affection and conviviality may appear to be friendly and giving, but they are often a desperate attempt to compensate for the profound feeling of joylessness within.

The Fire element gives us the capacity to love and be loved. In Western culture, the word 'love' is typically used to describe the way we feel about someone or something that triggers a heightened sense of wellbeing within us. In other words, it is conditional. In Taoist philosophy, love is not subject to any such conditions. On the contrary, it is the very force that gives rise to everything in the universe and, as such, it is not dependent on anything. To understand love, the physicians and philosophers of ancient China looked not to one other but to the natural world. What they saw was a perfectly balanced cycle of life, expanding and contracting in a never-ending sequence of creation and destruction that was unwavering and all-encompassing. Life itself was the ultimate expression of benevolence. To feel love, then, we need only surrender to the wonder and bliss of creation of which we are a part. In other words, we need only fall in love with ourselves, and it is the Fire element that enables us to do that.

* * *

On a sweltering Sunday afternoon in the middle of summer, I was alone in the clinic doing administrative work when I received a call from Jessie, asking if she could see me for an emergency appointment. She sounded distressed, so I told her to come right away. Half an hour later, the bell rang and I buzzed her in. I walked up to the waiting room and found her sitting in the dark with her head bowed. For a moment, I thought she was talking on her phone but then I realised that she was sobbing. I sat next to her and took her hand as the tears flowed. "Come on, Jessie, let's go downstairs." I put my arm around her shoulder and walked her slowly to my room. She sat on the edge of the armchair and stared at the floor while I gently closed the door. I pulled my chair close to hers and we sat in silence until the tears dried up.

"You need a new shirt, Gerad. That one's awful on you."

"What's going on, Jessie?"

"He left me."

"Who?"

"Chris. He ran away. Disappeared. Gone."

"I don't understand. When? Why?"

"Friday. We were having lunch together in Soho and we got into an argument. I was in a foul mood, partly because my period was so painful but mostly because Chris was being such a dick. I was pushing him to set aside some time to look at properties but he kept on finding reasons why we should wait and it was doing my head in, so I stupidly gave him an ultimatum. I told him that if he didn't get his act together then it was over between us."

"Did you mean it?"

"Of course not. I just wanted him to show some kind of commitment. I gave all of myself to him, you know? Anyway, he got all upset and stormed out of the restaurant. I had a hair appointment to go to but I couldn't get him off my mind. We'd had arguments before but something didn't feel right. I tried calling him as soon as I left the hair salon but his phone was going straight to voicemail, so I decided to go back to the flat. As I turned into Poland Street, I saw him walk out of our building and throw some bags into the back of a taxi. I shouted and ran after him but it was too late. The taxi took off and disappeared round the corner. I haven't seen him since."

"Oh my God, Jessie. Did he leave you a note? Something? Anything?"

"Nothing. He just packed a bag and left. I sat up all night, desperately hoping that he would call. Then in the early hours of the morning my phone lit up. Someone had withdrawn all of the funds from our savings account. That's when I knew he wasn't coming back. It's my worst nightmare. It's the most painful thing ever."

"Do you have any idea where he might have gone?"

"His brother called me this morning and told me that Chris had left the country but he wouldn't say where he'd gone. He said that he had a gambling addiction and had been using cocaine. Apparently he had run up huge debts and couldn't pay them off. I guess that's why he emptied our savings account. Everything we'd set aside to buy the house."

"You must be devastated, Jessie. It's hard to imagine."

"The worst thing is that I can't bring myself to tell anyone. It's just too embarrassing, and anyway, it's totally my fault that he left."

"Why on earth do you think it's your fault?"

"I put too much pressure on him. I'll regret it for the rest of my life."

We all get to choose how to frame the things that happen to us, but when someone breaks our heart, the sheer intensity of the experience can disable the rational mind. The explanation for Chris's disappearance had done nothing to lessen the pain that Jessie felt. Instead, she blamed herself. Being abandoned by the man she loved simply confirmed a long-held fear that she was unlovable.

PALACE OF WEARINESS

In the safety of my room, Jessie was able to function, but I was only too aware that once she left the clinic, this traumatic experience would weigh heavily on her. Having chosen not to tell anyone, she would be without support and would therefore be in a very vulnerable state. 'Spirit Gate' is a point on the Heart meridian located at the wrist. It is often used to treat shock, but my reason for choosing it that day was to re-establish the authority of the Heart official. The ancient Chinese pictured each person as a microcosm of Nature as a whole. 'Spirit Gate' is where the five spirits instate the authority of heaven over our individual lives. Any disturbance to this utopian environment, such as trauma or disease, causes the five spirits to take flight, resulting in the destabilisation of the person. After needling 'Spirit Gate', I could feel the twelve pulses come back into balance, which told me that Nature's authority had been reinstated.

* * *

Considering the extreme upheaval in her life, Jessie bounced back remarkably quickly, and before long she and Toto were back in my treatment room causing havoc.

"It's my birthday next week and the girls have planned a surprise for me. Please God don't let it be breakfast at the Firehouse."

"Do they know about Chris?"

"Yeah, everyone knows. My parents are over the moon and most of my friends think I'm better off without him. Thanks, everyone!"

"And how are you?" Jessie pulled her jacket tightly around her, which was her way of telling me that she was not up for talking about her feelings.

"I met someone in the park yesterday. Fabulous guy with a dreary wife."

"He told you his wife was dreary?"

"No, but you can tell. He was flirting outrageously with me even though I looked like an old bag lady." Jessie loved attention, particularly if it came from men, and she was very adept at attracting them. Even when she was with Chris, she was constantly surrounded by a string of admirers, but now that she was single, she was fighting them off with a stick. All she had to do was pick up her phone and they would flock to her doorstep, ready to whisk her off for a romantic weekend or a night at the theatre. Whether or not she really liked them was beside the point. It was all about being the centre of attention, and she was perfectly happy to let someone fall in love with her, even if she had absolutely no intention of returning the affection.

"What else? Let me see... Well, Daniel's taking me to New York for a long weekend."

"Daniel?"

"You know Daniel! I've told you about him a thousand times. He's the one who only comes up to my knees. He's been madly in love with me for years."

"So why are you going to New York with him?"

"He makes me laugh and he treats me like a princess." She thrust her phone at me to show me a picture of her and Daniel from some bygone era. It was as if she wanted me to know that she was lovable.

"The footballer's been in touch, too."

"The one who never cheats on his wife?"

"Exactly. He's asked me to meet him in Paris." She winked at me and then burst into laughter. "I tell you, they're all coming out of the woodwork now." Jessie's excitement was palpable. She was clearly having a whale of a time and I could feel myself getting caught up in the excitement, yet I couldn't help wondering what was really going on behind all the fun and games. Was she really alright? What was it about the state of her Fire element that enabled her to shift so rapidly from heartbreak to frivolity? As happy as I was to see her so full of joy, I was also very aware that when the light burns so brightly it can often be a sign of its imminent demise. From a treatment perspective, it was clear that the fire within her was feeding on the oxygen of external stimuli, and would only survive if it had a solid foundation from which to draw its strength. That day, I chose the Water point on the Circulation-Sex official to temper any excess fire, after which I added the Wood points on both Fire meridians to gently feed the flame at its source. As I finished reading her pulses, Jessie gently gripped my hand. The officials seemed to be expressing their gratitude for a renewed sense of warmth and care.

For the next couple of months, Jessie poured all of her energy into her work, her friends and her increasingly colourful love life. She came to see me weekly and soon reported pain-free periods with no abnormal bleed. But there was something else that troubled me. She had a lump on one of her breasts that her doctor had dismissed as a cyst, but she also told me that she had been feeling unusually tired and had a persistent pain in one of her arms. I advised her to see her doctor again as soon as possible and insist on a check. A couple of weeks later, I was clearing up my room at the end of a long day when I received a text from her.

"Lump is not a cyst. Had biopsy. Waiting for results. YIKES!"

I sent her a reassuring voice message but ten days later, I got another text.

"Bad news… I need to see you."

Jessie came in early the following morning. She looked scared. "It's the big C. They want me to have a double mastectomy."

"Oh, Jessie. I don't know what to say."

"Don't worry, I'm not doing it. I've said yes to chemo but that's it. I'd rather die with my boobs intact than spend the rest of my life stuffing socks in my bra."

We spent some time talking about the decisions she would have to make regarding her care, but the thing she was most afraid of was not being in control. I had already seen how carefully she had crafted the narrative after Chris abandoned her and she was doing the very same thing now. "I'll survive this, I know I will. But I'll do it my way. I'm not telling anyone and I told the cancer nurse that I don't want any sympathy. If they treat me like a victim, I'm outta there."

"I will do my very best to help you through this, Jessie."

"I know you will, thank you. My oncologist, Ezra, is amazing, too. He totally gets me."

Over the next few weeks, Jessie adjusted to her new reality with fearless determination and characteristic humour, but something about her had changed. The relationship with her oncologist seemed to have ignited something in her, and I couldn't help noticing the way she blushed when I asked her about him. She insisted that their relationship was entirely professional, but there was definitely a frisson in the air whenever his name was mentioned.

"He's trying to persuade me to have the mastectomy. He says I'll be beautiful with or without breasts but I'm not convinced. They're part of me, you know? They're part of what makes me a woman."

It was not my place to advise Jessie on the pros and cons of surgery, but I knew that her ability to make the right decision in any area of her life was dependent to a large extent on how balanced she was in body, mind and spirit. If she was in a state of equilibrium, she would intuitively know what was best for her. If not, her decisions would likely be reactionary. All I could do was support her officials in the hope that she would see what was best for her.

* * *

The next time Jessie came to see me, she was dressed in a figure-hugging pink tracksuit. She sashayed across the room, turned her head from side to side like a model on the catwalk and then spun around to face me. "You see? That weight loss point does work." She slumped into the chair and let out a long, weary sigh.

"What's going on, Jessie?"

"Someone told me that Chris had been in town. It really shook me." For a moment, I thought she was going to burst into tears but she composed herself and started scrolling through her phone. "Do you know who Maya Angelou is?"

"The poet?" She tossed her phone into my lap and looked away.

"'*Love recognises no barriers. It jumps hurdles, leaps fences, penetrates walls to arrive at its destination full of hope.*' That's beautiful, Jessie. Does that express the way you're feeling?"

"Had you asked me that a few months ago, I would have said no, but I feel hopeful again for the first time since Chris left me."

"What's changed?"

She blushed and pulled the hood of her tracksuit over her eyes like a shy child. "Something strange happened the other day. I was at the hospital with Ezra and, while we were talking, he put his hand on my forearm and left it there. I felt this intense heat radiating up my arm and into my chest. It was as if my heart was opening up like a flower. I felt weirdly exposed but there was a sense of safety and relief as well. I feel happy."

"One of my friends calls it the touch of human kindness. There's not enough of that around. But Jessie, he's your oncologist. Be careful."

Personal and professional boundaries are an essential part of the patient/practitioner relationship. In the Five-Element tradition, we are taught that love is the source of all creation and, as such, it plays a fundamental role in the healing process, but how can the practitioner work from a place of love without creating a merging or dependent relationship? Patients respond to warmth and care in different ways. Most people see their practitioner as just that, but others will project a persona or an imagined relationship onto them, so it is essential to maintain clear parameters. I was delighted to see Jessie in such an upbeat mood but I was also worried. Was she beginning to see her oncologist as the person who could give her the intimacy and love she craved? If so, she was likely playing with fire.

The aim of the treatment that day was to support her natural capacity to be open and receive the care she needed, while maintaining healthy boundaries. I started with two points on the back, which go directly to the Fire officials and give them all the encouragement and energy they need to perform their unique roles. I then chose two spirit points: 'Gate of Qi Reserve' provides an energetic pit stop for repair and renewal, while 'Assembly of Ancestors' enables the officials to tap into our inherent wisdom, which is passed down from one generation to the next.

The following week, Jessie strode into my treatment room with a mischievous grin on her face.

"Can you keep a secret, Gerad?"

"Of course."

"I've been seeing someone."
"That's wonderful! Who's the lucky man?"
"Ezra."

The confirmation of this inappropriate relationship left me speechless. How had Jessie's emotional pendulum swung from one extreme to another in such a short time? The shift from the vulnerable and frightened woman who had showed up on the first day of treatment to the calm and confident woman before me now was remarkable. However, I knew only too well how many of my patients with a Causative Factor in Fire would light up with the arrival of a new project or plaything, only to fade once the initial euphoria had dissipated.

"Are you sure this is wise, Jessie? He's your oncologist. And he's married, no?"

"Technically, yes, but it's not going to last. They're always arguing and they never have sex. Anyway, this is the most important thing for me right now."

In ancient Chinese philosophy, the Fire element was given an elevated status for two important reasons. Firstly, it was seen as the element most closely related to heaven. Fire was represented by the sun, radiating its life-giving energy from above. Secondly, when mapping the human body to understand the network of meridians, the Chinese discovered that the Fire element had two functional officials (Circulation-Sex and Three Heater) in addition to those relating to the physical organs (the Heart and the Small Intestine). The Heart official is likened to the ruler of an Empire, with the Small Intestine official as its loyal envoy. Supporting them are the Circulation-Sex and Three

Heater officials, which are responsible for disseminating and regulating warmth and passion, as well as managing the communication between all of the officials. So many of the things we associate with being a passionate, warm-blooded human, such as intimacy, communication, fun and sex, are under the jurisdiction of these officials. The Circulation-Sex official is known as the heart protector. When this official functions in harmony with Nature's design, we are able to manage our relationships in a balanced and healthy manner. When it doesn't, we tend to lose sight of appropriate boundaries and place ourselves in emotional jeopardy.

* * *

Jessie continued with the chemotherapy and, to my dismay, also continued seeing Ezra. But all was not well, and although she managed to project a cheerful persona in public, the cracks were beginning to show. It wasn't long before a request for an urgent appointment arrived once again in my inbox. When she showed up at the clinic, her energy was palpably low. Even Toto seemed to have lost his usual spark.

"The chemo isn't working. It's messing with my bone marrow, so I've got to lay off the treatment for a while. Ezra doesn't seem to know what's going on, so I'm hoping you can do something." Jessie's manner was casual, but I could tell from her demeanour that she had taken a knock. This was the first setback since her cancer treatment began and it was clearly troubling her.

"I'll do my best. My goal is to keep you as balanced as possible on every level. That way your body will be as fit as it can be to face whatever the illness throws at you. I can also do a point called 'Rich for the Vitals', which boosts bone marrow production."

"Thank you, Gerad, I don't know what I would do without you."

"How are things with Ezra? Are you managing to juggle being a patient and a lover at the same time?" Although Jessie immediately tried to change the subject, I persevered. I was teasing her, but given my concerns about the ethical issues involved in her medical care, I genuinely wanted to know the answer.

"We're doing just fine."

"I've got to be honest, Jessie, I think it would be much better if you asked to be transferred to a different consultant. Not only is it unethical for Ezra to be in a sexual relationship with you, it's also essential for a medical professional to maintain objectivity."

"Nonsense! You and I are friends and it's never affected the treatments, has it?" The relationship with Ezra seemed to fulfil an important need for Jessie at this difficult time, but what she really needed was to find the naturally occurring joy inside herself.

I started the treatment that day with 'Dovetail', which is located at the centre of the abdomen, just below the small bone that sits at the bottom of the rib cage. It is at this location that the energy rises and fills the chest region, enabling us to stand tall and cope with the ups and downs of life. The 'dove' in the name derives from the two lobes of the lungs, which are like the spreading wings of a bird, while the 'tail' relates to an outward expression of joy from the heart, like the wagging tail of a dog. It's a common misconception that our happiness depends on external conditions. The truth is that they mirror something that already exists within us.

Five burning moxa to warm the point and a stimulating needle action on Dovetail immediately restored a pinkish tone to Jessie's complexion and a sense of ease to the room. Toto felt it immediately. He jumped down from the treatment couch, settled into my chair and nodded off. I continued with 'Rich for the Vitals' and ended with two more points on the Fire meridians called 'Inner and Outer Frontier Gate'. The 'Gates' enable us to know instinctively when to open our hearts to the outer world and when to retreat to the safety of our inner sanctum.

A week later, Jessie came for a follow-up appointment. As I walked up the stairs to collect her, I could already hear her laughter coming from the waiting room. As I reached the top of the staircase, Toto sprinted past me with a silk scarf in his mouth, an irate Eszter in hot pursuit. She managed to corner him, but as she snatched the scarf from his teeth, there was a loud tearing noise. Toto stood at the end of the corridor looking sheepish, the remnants of Eszter's scarf in his mouth.

"I tell you, Gerad, one of these days I'm going to do something illegal to that dog. He's completely out of control. As is his owner."

I walked into the waiting room to find Jessie lying on

her back on one of the sofas, wrapped in an ankle-length puffer jacket. She had removed her boots and was making circles in the air with one of her feet. As always, she was on the phone.

"Gotta run. Gerad's here." She slid her boots on, gathered up her things and grinned at me. "Have you seen Toto?"

"Yup, he's out here playing with Eszter." I winked at Eszter, who scowled at me and muttered something under her breath. Jessie grabbed Toto and attached the lead to his collar.

"What have you got in your mouth? Drop it!" She removed a piece of sodden fabric from his mouth and inspected it. "Ugh! That's disgusting! Where did you find that?" She tossed it into the bin by Eszter's desk and headed off in the direction of my room. I followed her downstairs, pulled her notes from the filing cabinet and waited for her to settle. She dropped into one of the armchairs with a thud and started showering Toto with kisses.

"So, how are you, Jessie?"

"Well, let's see. Chris ran away with all my money, I've got cancer and Ezra just dumped me."

"Really?"

"Yes, really."

"Dare I ask why?"

"Oh, I don't know. Because he's a man? Now that he's had his way with me he's suddenly decided that it's inappropriate to be in a relationship with one of his patients. He told me it's his duty to focus on my recovery."

PALACE OF WEARINESS

"What did you say?"

"I told him it's his duty to fuck off."

"Fair enough."

"I should have seen it coming. After our last session, I left here feeling really strong and confident. I spent the evening with him and I suddenly saw him in a different light. He was all insecure and needy and he kept on saying how guilty he felt for cheating on his wife. Then he says, 'From now on when you come for an appointment you've got to come as my patient, not as my lover.' I said, 'I *am* your fucking patient!' Then on Thursday he asked me to meet him at the end of his shift and he told me that he was going to refer me to a different consultant. He said it was for the best. That was his way of saying that it was over between us. It was all so cold and matter of fact. Men can be such arseholes, you know? I don't want any more of them in my life. You and Toto, that's it."

"Maybe it's for the best, Jessie. The most important thing right now is your recovery."

"Maybe. But it hurts. Anyway, it's OK. I'm OK. Really."

Despite the rejection, there was something rather majestic about Jessie that day. It felt as though she had risen above it all, that she had taken back control of her destiny. In recent months, the impact of the chemotherapy had taken its toll on her, but the radiant quality of her spirit had returned and her voice was rich and strong. "I'm gonna beat this thing, Gerad. I'm gonna give it my all now." Jessie's resolve to take responsibility for her health was heartening, but I was still aware of an underlying sadness and fragility. My concern was that if she didn't fully invest in this renewed sense of strength and her determination to survive, things could quickly fall apart.

"What do you need right now, Jessie?

"I need to exorcise that spineless little weasel from every cell in my body and learn the lesson."

"What would that lesson be?"

"To stop chasing these pathetic, narcissistic men."

"And your part in all of this?"

"I guess I'm always looking for the next shiny object that will brighten up my day. I've always done it. I put so much energy into all of my relationships but as much as I enjoy them, I often end up feeling resentful and hurt. I've had enough."

'Palace of Weariness' was the perfect point for Jessie at this pivotal moment. I remembered times in my own life when I was exhausted from trying to keep the show on the road, feeling responsible for everyone else's happiness when all I wanted was to pull back and retreat. 'Palace of Weariness' is the key to our own private oasis, a sacred inner space where we can retreat and bask in the warm glow of the love that naturally resides within each and every one of us. It's like the most perfect boutique hotel in which everything is designed to satisfy our own unique needs and desires. Whenever we open our heart to someone we take a risk. This beautiful point gives us the strength to step into the uncharted waters of love and romance, aware of its pitfalls but open to its rewards.

PALACE OF WEARINESS

* * *

In the months that followed, Jessie remained relatively stable but I noticed a gradual decline in her energy and, in particular, a shortness of breath. Her doctor put it down to anaemia, but I was worried that the cancer might have spread. She managed to maintain her natural exuberance, but while she talked at length about her plans for the future, she also became increasingly nostalgic, reminiscing about the busy, glamorous life that she used to have. She had scaled back her work to the bare minimum, and when she wasn't at the hospital, she spent most of her time at home with Toto, calling her friends one after the other until late into the evening. One day, she arrived for her session and slumped in the chair without uttering a word. There was a distinct air of resignation about her.

"What's going on, Jessie?"

"It just feels so hopeless sometimes. I don't want to give up but the odds seem to be stacked against me." I took her hand, returning the familiar squeeze that she so often gave me as she left the clinic. Toto, sensing her sadness, jumped onto the chair and settled beside her. Jessie was clearly on a low ebb, but even in her darkest moments, I could always sense the optimism that lay just beneath the surface. Even though the fire in her belly that had been ignited after she and Ezra ended their affair might have diminished somewhat, I knew that as long as the embers were glowing, there was still hope that it could burn brightly once again. Emboldened by my understanding of the workings of Nature and in particular the nature of the Fire element, I set aside any thoughts of defeat and focused on the balance of the elements that constituted this courageous woman.

"Right! Onto the couch, madam. Boots off, top off, phone off. We're going to build the most stunningly beautiful fire that Nature ever made." As always, I employed a treatment strategy that followed natural law. Transfers of energy from any of the elements that had a relative excess were directed to the Fire. Points that would encourage the Fire to burn were warmed and needled. Finally, supportive points that would create the necessary environment for the flames to gather strength were stimulated. Five days later, Jessie was back in the room.

"Holy shit! What did you do to me? I felt so horny, I almost ate the postman alive. Anyway, you'll be glad to hear that I managed to restrain my animal impulses and I've been channelling the energy into looking after myself."

"I'm delighted to hear that. How's your week been?"

"Wonderful! After our last session, I couldn't stop giggling. Everything seemed so bizarre and funny but weirdly I didn't feel the urge to call anyone and share the fun like I normally do. I was just happy to enjoy it all on my own. The next morning while I was waiting for the coffee to brew, I grabbed a wooden spoon and started joking around like I was on the stage. It's what I used to do when I was a kid. I used to spend hours practising a stand-up comedy routine in front of my bedroom mirror and then I'd put on a show for my friends at school.

Everyone thought I was really funny." As soon as she started talking about her passion for comedy, her eyes lit up. The contrast between the sad, wounded woman and the bright, mischievous girl who loved to make people laugh was striking.

"Why did you give it up?"

"Shame, I guess. During one of the school holidays I did a show for my family and some of my parents' friends. Later that day, my father took me aside and told me that I should stop showing off. He said no man wants a wife who makes a fool of herself. I felt so embarrassed."

"Well, for what it's worth, I think you would make a great comedian." Throughout her life, Jessie had yearned to love and be loved, but she had always looked to others to fulfil that desire. Now, finally, she was beginning to understand that the person she needed to fall in love with was herself. The talented, funny, charismatic girl who had been extinguished all those years ago seemed to have risen from the ashes. My job now was to ensure that the bright and exciting force that was emerging within her would endure and sweep away any obstacles that might stand in the way of her recovery and rebirth.

It's easy to buy into the generally fatalistic Western view of illness, but what we forget is that the human body, mind and spirit are always actively seeking restoration of the natural order. Anything that disturbs this instinctive movement back to wholeness is a cause of disease. From a Five-Element perspective, the original cause of Jessie's condition was an imbalance in the Fire element, which prevented the other officials from maintaining their normal functions, creating an unstable and chaotic environment.

Amongst other things, the officials of the Fire element are responsible for the regulation of temperature, which is essential for healthy cell division and an overall sense of harmony between the officials. The Fire element brings warmth, light and a transformative power to our lives, as well as passion, enthusiasm and healing. The fundamental purpose of any living organism is to survive and reproduce, but humans have evolved to such a degree that our purpose can be more exalted than this. Once we give our full attention to what really fills us with passion and joy, the magic starts to happen.

Jessie's transformation was astonishing. Within weeks, she had written a one-woman show and was busy getting gigs to try it out. I went to see her perform in a pub in Hampstead and I was blown away by her gift for entertaining a crowd. Her health concerns seemed to have been replaced by a profound sense of excitement and happiness. Then, a few months later, she booked in for an urgent appointment. She appeared to be cheerful but something was clearly troubling her.

"Jessie? What's up?"

"I got my latest scan results. The tumours in my liver have doubled in size, despite the new trial I've been on. I've been feeling a strange sensation under my rib cage. I knew something was wrong." I froze. I had suspected that her prognosis was not good but the confirmation hit me hard. Jessie was more than just a patient. She felt like family and the prospect of losing her affected me deeply.

"How are you processing this new development?"

"There's a strong chance I could die, I guess." I stayed very still, focusing entirely on her concerns rather than my own. My training and all my years in practice had taught me repeatedly that my role is to be an 'instrument of Nature'. I desperately wanted Jessie to survive, but even thinking that I could interfere with her destiny would be wrong. My responsibility was to be honest and mirror the courage that she had shown throughout her ordeal.

"Have you really taken on board that this could be it, Jessie?"

"I've told a few people what's going on but they all seem to think they have the answer. Cancer clinics in eastern Europe, rhino's feet, all that stuff." Jessie began to tear up. Her voice had become flat and lifeless and she looked defeated.

"I think you should see me weekly from now on. Is that OK with you?" We looked at each other knowingly. Even though were both fully aware of the charade, neither of us wanted to let go of whatever shred of optimism remained.

"I would love that, thank you."

There was a limit to what I could hope to do for Jessie, but as summer was once again in full swing, I decided to treat the Fire points on the Fire officials' meridians. If there were to be a miracle from treatment, it would be through these points. Two days later, Jessie emailed me to say that the treatment had helped and asked if she could arrange her appointments for the coming months. I replied with suggested dates but, surprisingly, she couldn't fit most of them into her schedule. Pilates, personal training, lunch dates and even a new manager were taking up most of her time. Her optimism and enthusiasm for life never ceased to amaze me. Even in her darkest moments she had a fervent desire to fill her life with purpose and joy. Jessie cancelled our last scheduled appointment with a voice message.

Hi darling, I'm really not good. I'm back in hospital and they say I'll be here for a few days. They've got to drain the fluid from my kidneys but don't worry about me. The girls are here and we're planning a trip to Barbados.

Jessie died a week later. Her mother called to thank me for being a good friend to her daughter. Losing her was heartbreaking. I saw so much of myself in her. Being her practitioner while managing all the personal triggers that challenged my professional role was a struggle. Thankfully, my experience of working with people has taught me that the love and affection we inherently have for each other supersedes any formalised or professional relationship.

9

WALK BETWEEN

*

From: Ella Tesfay
To: Kite Clinic
Good morning. Please book me with Gerad Kite next week. I am only available at the following times: Tuesday 10.15, Thursday 14.00, Friday 17.00
  Ella

From: Kite Clinic
To: Ella Tesfay
Hi Ella,
Thanks for your interest in treatment with me. The first availability I have for a new patient is in three weeks. I can offer you 10am on Wed 25th May. I look forward to hearing from you.
  Best wishes
  Gerad Kite

From: Ella Tesfay
To: Kite Clinic
I already explained that I need to be seen next week.

Please read my first email or have someone call me.

From: Kite Clinic
To: Ella Tesfay
Hi Ella,
The first availability I have for a new patient is 25th May but if you need to be seen urgently I could squeeze you in next Wednesday at 8am.
  Best wishes
  Gerad

From: Ella Tesfay
To: Kite Clinic
OK

* * *

Ella's arrival was dramatic. I walked into the waiting room, curious to meet the author of the feisty emails, only to find Eszter standing by the window with her face pressed up against the glass.

"What's going on, Eszter? You told me my patient was here." Eszter turned to face me, leaving an abstract impression of her face on the steamed-up glass.

"She was but then she spotted the warden." I joined Eszter at the window and looked out onto the street below. Directly in front of the clinic was a silver Mercedes with a parking ticket on the windscreen. Beside it, a smartly dressed woman was wagging her finger angrily at a red-faced traffic warden in an ill-fitting uniform. He was clearly trying to explain why he had given her a ticket and she was clearly having none of it. The words flew out of her mouth like bullets from a gun, rat-a-tat-tat, and the poor man shuffled a little further backwards as each one found its target. She ripped the ticket from beneath the windscreen wiper, tore it in half and handed it to her browbeaten victim before marching back to the clinic. I walked into the hallway and opened the front door just as she reached the top of the steps.

"Horrible little man. How dare he!" She brushed past me, removed a piece of paper from her handbag and slapped it on Eszter's desk. "Right, let's try again. I have an appointment with Mr Kite. Here's the email."

Eszter put on her glasses and peered at the print-out. "So you do. Well, Mr Kite is right behind you."

The woman spun round and scanned me from head to toe. "Why didn't you say so?" She gripped my hand and shook it vigorously. "Right, let's get on with it! It's this way, I presume." She walked down the corridor and waited for me by the stairs. "Up? Down? Straight ahead?"

"Down. Let me lead the way."

We walked downstairs in lock step without saying a word, but every time she grabbed the handrail I could hear the jingling of her bangles and the sharp rap of her rings as they made contact with the wood. I opened the door to my room and ushered her in. She swept past me, removed her jacket and handed it to me before sitting down in my chair. I hung it on the back of the door and politely asked her to change places. She switched chairs, crossed her legs and cleared her throat in a manner that made her irritation obvious.

"Happy now?"

Ella was a tall, willowy woman in her late thirties who scared the life out of all but her most robust adversaries. She dressed immaculately in dark suits and high-heeled shoes that she would absent-mindedly click together, echoing the staccato rhythm of her speech. She had been born in Berlin, the eldest daughter of Ethiopian immigrants who had fled the country after war broke out with Somalia in the late seventies. From a young age, it was clear that she was academically gifted, and by seventeen, she had won a place at the London School of Economics. After graduating, she decided to stay and began working for one of the tech giants. Five years later, she was headhunted by an AI start-up and was now earning a huge salary as chief financial officer. She had a large apartment overlooking Regent's Park and a lifestyle that belonged in a magazine. Unfortunately, she was miserable. While she was still at school, she had mapped out a plan for her life: work hard in her twenties, meet a man when she was twenty-eight, get married at thirty, have her first child at thirty-two. They would spend the week in a townhouse and retire to the countryside for weekends. It was the perfect plan but it hadn't materialised and she was furious. The moment she sat down in the chair opposite me, I knew that I had met my match. Everything about her spoke of someone who meant business. The way she dressed, the way she sat, the way she spoke, the way she looked at me. It might have been my clinic, but as far as she was concerned, there was only one person in charge and it wasn't me.

"Welcome, Ella. I'm sorry you had a bit of a bumpy start this morning."

"Bumpy? Believe me, that's nothing."

"OK, well let's get started then, shall we?" I started to explain how I work but was quickly interrupted.

"Please, I don't need all the fluff. I've read your book. What's it called? Making Babies?"

"The Art of Baby Making."

"That's the one. So, let's cut to the chase. I'm thirty-nine, I'm single and I don't have any children. I don't need help finding a man but I do need to ensure that I remain fertile until I do."

"Thank you for reading my book. You will have gathered in that case that I need to carry out a full investigation for the purpose of diagnosis." I found myself matching her no-nonsense manner of speaking. It was an involuntary reflex but it was telling. And effective. She uncrossed her legs and straightened her spine.

"What do you want to know?"

"As you suggested, let's focus on why you're here. To start with, let's talk about your menstrual health and any medical investigations you've had relating to your fertility."

"Well, my periods started when I was thirteen and they're as regular as clockwork. On day ten I get copious amounts of cervical mucus, which continues for five days. My temperature rises during ovulation and the twenty-eight day bleed is heavy and painful for five days."

She glowered at me triumphantly. "And my fertility tests showed that everything is working perfectly."

"That's great news, Ella. Let's talk about the missing link. Are you in a relationship?"

"No! I already told you that."

"You're right, you did just tell me that, I'm sorry." I felt like I had just been told off by the teacher for not paying attention. One more misstep and I would be told to stand in the corner. I uncrossed my legs to mirror her posture and leaned in towards her. "Have you had any long-term relationships?"

"Yes."

"How many?"

"Two."

"Could you tell me about them?"

"Why?" I found it hard to conceal my frustration and Ella noticed. "Look, I'm not trying to be difficult. I just want you to get on and fix my 'jing' or whatever it is you do." During these kinds of encounters, it can be hard to distinguish between my personal reactions to patients and useful diagnostic information. The interaction had become adversarial and I was feeling under pressure to treat her before I had even made a diagnosis. Just as I was about to throw in the towel, a flash of green around her temples caught my eye. Nature was reminding me where I needed to focus my attention. It was time to pull Ella back into line and continue with the job in hand.

"Ella, this is what we're going to do. We're going to talk about your history and then we'll get on with the treatment." Had I known what was about to unfold, I might have run while I had the chance, but the ensuing rant actually served an important purpose. By the time it was finished, my diagnosis was almost complete. She began by roasting Carl, the first boyfriend with whom she had tried to have children. They were still great friends but as a partner he had been useless. He had pursued her for months, she said, spinning her a yarn about his career ambitions and his desire to have a family, but it was all a pipe dream. When he failed to propose, Ella decided to skip the marriage part and start trying for a baby right away, but as soon as she came off the pill, Carl developed erectile dysfunction.

"He's a lovely guy but I had to move on. I'm clear about what I want in life and I need a partner who can help me achieve that." Next up was Hakeem, the man she had thought was the love of her life. They met on a friend's boat in the south of France when she was thirty-four and they quickly became inseparable. Within six months, they were living together and not long afterwards Hakeem proposed to her. "I explained clearly and carefully that I needed to get the plan back on track and start a family immediately. We tried for a while but nothing happened, so I decided to use a fertility clinic. I had four good embryos from two rounds of IVF but none of them even produced a pregnancy, let alone a baby."

"You didn't mention IVF when I asked about your fertility history. Did they tell you why they thought the embryos hadn't implanted?"

"No, but it's obvious."

"Really?"

"Yes! Some men have strong genes. Hakeem doesn't."
"So you called off the engagement?"
"Yes."
"Are you still friends with him, too?"
"Of course. I don't believe in burning bridges. He's a great dinner companion, as is Carl." The demolition continued. Carl and Hakeem were followed by a long list of former friends and colleagues who had failed to live up to the mark. Anyone who got in the way of her life plan had been summarily dispatched. I was now in little doubt that her Causative Factor was in the Wood element. The green colour to the side of her eyes was as vivid as can be, and the emotion that filled the room was tangible. Everything she said had an angry charge to it, and it was hard not to be intimidated. Then there was the sound in her voice, the persistent, rhythmic clip of a barking dog. Nevertheless, until I had all four legs of the stool, I couldn't be absolutely certain of my diagnosis. I still needed to confirm her odour.

"OK, Ella, on the treatment couch please. Shoes off, shirt off, please. I'll be back in a second." I left the room to wash my hands, but when I came back, she was still in the chair with her legs crossed. "Is everything OK?"

"Why do I have to take my shirt off?"

"Because I need your back for the first treatment. Does that make you uncomfortable?" She took a deep breath and exhaled sharply to release her irritation.

"A little, yes, but so be it." She removed her satin shirt and strode past me to lie down on the treatment couch. As she did so, I caught the familiar odour of soured milk in her wake. My diagnosis was complete. It was indeed the Wood element that was calling for help. I picked up her hand to feel the pulses and was immediately struck by the stiffness in her arm. I shook it gently to see if I could release the tension, but she responded by gripping my hand and tightening her forearm. The fingers on her other hand were splayed out, taut and unbending, and her eyes were fixed on the ceiling.

As with all first treatments on the Wood element, I needled the source points of the Liver and Gallbladder officials. As the needles connected with the points, Ella relaxed and her eyes closed. I took her pulses again and was happy to note that the energy shared by the five elements had evened out. The tension had all but dissipated from her arms and her fingers had returned to a resting position. When she swung her legs over the edge of the treatment couch and walked over to her chair to gather her things, her movements were fluid and graceful. It was a marked difference from the brittle, pugnacious woman who had marched into the room an hour earlier.

* * *

Ella arrived for her second treatment twenty minutes late, so I asked Eszter to send her down right away. There was no apology. She simply plonked herself down in the armchair and slapped her knees with the palms of her hands. "Right, let's talk about your treatment. I felt very calm for about forty-eight hours, which I assume was your intention, but my period was due the day after and it still hasn't come. I don't know how you managed to mess up my cycle but you did, so I need you to fix that."

Human behaviour has been the fascination of physicians and philosophers alike since time immemorial. Why are we the way we are? Is it nature or nurture? Can we change our personality or is it fixed? Part of the beauty of the Five-Element philosophy is its simplicity. Through their close observation of the natural world and human behaviour, the ancient Chinese concluded that we are an integral part of Nature and, as such, we are subject to her immutable cycles and laws. Contrary to many theories of behaviour, they believed that the way that we manifest in this world is not down to our own volition. Each of us, they maintained, is an expression of Nature, the unique and inevitable outcome of the five elements and their associated officials. Ella's belligerent manner was not the result of people or things standing in the way of what she wanted to achieve at any given moment. That was simply the way she perceived the world. But if parking attendants and other assorted annoyances weren't the problem, what was it? Seen through the lens of Five-Element theory, the answer was simple. The part of her that would enable her to navigate her life with ease, grace and flexibility was in trouble. The shout in her voice and the feeling of anger that filled the room were not inherently hers. They were the outward signs of an inner imbalance.

The season of spring demonstrates everything we need to know about the Wood element and its unique gifts. As we emerge from the still depths of winter, Nature bursts into life with youthful vigour and unstoppable force. "Have another go!" she shouts, as the new cycle begins. This rallying cry gives us a profound sense of hope and excitement. Once again, the potential for change is ours. But while the possibility of rebirth is embodied so perfectly by the spring, it is not limited to that season. The qualities of the Wood element are ever present within us. Each and every second of our life we have an opportunity to grow. In a state of balance, this natural capacity enables us to live life with the grace and freedom of a bird drifting on warm currents of air. When the Wood element is compromised, however, we feel restricted and frustrated. Every day is a struggle, and rather than allow ourselves to be carried by the wind, we fight it head-on until we collapse in exhaustion and resignation.

The Liver official is considered to be the general of the armed forces, whose role is to weigh up the situation and make plans accordingly. Like a commander on the battlefield, we all need to be able to see our goals in life and have a strategy in place that will enable us to achieve them. According to the Taoist tradition, each of us has a blueprint that is contained within the Kidney official, but we are neither destined nor designed to be limited by it. On the contrary, all of us have the freedom to adjust our sights as we move through life, and it is the Wood element that gives us this capacity. Without it, we lose the vitality and freshness of our existence. We become stuck and angry at our inability to move forward and achieve what we instinctively know we are capable of. I hadn't known Ella for long, but it was obvious to me that the struggle to realise her dreams was born of a complete lack of flexibility, the result of her tunnel vision. Like so many of us, she wanted a partner, a home, a family and a career, but rather than allow life to unfold naturally, she expected it to fall in line with her rigid and immovable plan. There was no room for anyone or anything to be other than the way she expected. She had life in a stranglehold and she was trying to choke it into submission. When she walked into my room that morning and accused me of messing up her menstrual cycle, it was a little hard to take, but the accusation was designed to challenge me, so I picked up the gauntlet without hesitation.

"It's most likely that your cycle is recalibrating. Many women have a regular twenty-eight-day cycle that is out of sync with other cycles in the body. It may just be that yours is adjusting to a new start and end date. Let's see when it comes, shall we?"

"Interesting." She narrowed her eyes and forced a half smile. After the slight misstep in our first meeting, I felt like I had been put on a warning, but it seemed that I had redeemed myself. Perhaps I wouldn't have to stand in the corner after all?

"Ella, time is precious. I'd like to crack on with the treatment right away, so please remove your shoes and tights while I wash my hands."

Generally, I spend twenty minutes or so at the beginning of each session asking patients about their week or learning more about their life, but on this occasion I wasn't convinced that talking was going to tell me anything I didn't already know. My relationship with Ella had already been established and it felt unnecessary, perhaps even provocative, to trap her in the chair and grill her. Ultimately, in the practice of Five-Element Acupuncture, the most important communication is that between the practitioner and the officials, and that happens via the medium of the needles. Many people find it difficult to believe that we can stimulate a so-called point with a sharp object and deliver an outcome. Indeed, such scepticism is understandable if one cannot think of one's own essence as anything other than a physical form. In Western terms, the liver is a physical organ that filters blood and breaks down poisonous substances such as alcohol and drugs. For the ancient Chinese, the organs of the body were seen as the physical manifestation of the officials, which also govern the domains of the mind and the spirit. The way they saw it, the Liver official incorporated not only the organ but also a meridian pathway, the nails, the eyes and all of the attributes that we associate with the Wood element on every level of our being. As general of the armed forces, the Liver official's role is to assess the field of battle and prepare the plan for its foot soldiers to execute. So when practitioners needle a point, they are tapping into a field of energy that responds to stimuli and produces an effect in all three domains of our existence. My brief interaction with Ella that morning had been telling. It was clear that she needed a sparring partner and it appeared that she considered me to be a sufficiently worthy opponent. It was only by bouncing off someone that she would be able to find the strength to release herself from the bondage of her self-created limitations and reach up to the sky. Nature was telling me to reinvigorate this natural capacity for growth within her.

'Supreme Rushing' is the third point on the Liver official and it gives us a sense of freedom and expansion. It is likened to the mole emerging from its long hibernation and rushing out into the spring sunshine. Ella believed she was free but it was an illusion. Far from liberating her, her rigid plans and beliefs trapped her in a cage of her own making, tightly bound by intransigence and conceit. She was right about everything. Why couldn't everyone else see that? When her plan didn't materialise, rather than review it to see if it needed to yield in some way, she simply doubled down and applied more force. Ella's appointment that day started late and finished early. She seemed pleased with my efficiency, and as she left the room, she turned to thank me with an openness and generosity that took me by surprise. We were doing well.

* * *

Treatment number three began at eight o'clock sharp. By now there was an unspoken agreement between us. The sessions would start and finish on time, our verbal interaction would be short and to the point and the treatment would be efficient and effective.

"How are you, Ella?"

"Good question. So, first of all, I've been feeling relaxed just like last time, which is all very nice except that being laid back is *not* what I need. The clock is ticking and there are things I want to achieve. Secondly, I screwed something up at work, which was not funny. I don't make mistakes. Please do *not* do that to me again!"

Ella's manner was still brusque but there was no malign intent. It was simply an expression of the overwhelming frustration that gnawed away at her day after day. When the Wood element fails in its remit to design and execute a viable plan for life, we lose our sense of hope and can come across as grumpy and cross. This was very much my experience of Ella. Nevertheless, there was something different about her that morning. As punchy as she still was, there was a softening in our interaction. It now felt more like a collaboration than a confrontation and there was even room for a touch of humour.

"I won't do that again, Ella. I promise." Ella noticed my smile. She was smart enough to know that it wasn't in my power to put her to sleep and my submissive retort was understood by her as it was intended. We both knew that change was afoot and that tripping up at work, although unfortunate, was a positive sign. She was human after all. "You've got to break eggs to make omelettes," I told her.

"OK, let's break some more," she replied.

It had already become clear to me that much of Ella's irritability stemmed from her determination to force her plan into being by any means necessary. Now was the time to help her Liver official remember that although strength and assertion are needed to move forward in life, we also need the capacity to yield when necessary. 'Walk Between' is the second point on the Liver meridian. The Chinese character depicts two large wooden doors which have been shut tight, preventing anything from entering or leaving, but on one of the doors is a thin crack through which light passes. The light represents our innate ability to overcome the obstacles that stand in our way by choosing the path of least resistance. For the Chinese, the image of 'Walk Between' was of an advancing army, which automatically adjusts its formation to pass through a narrow gorge. In Nature we see the same reflex as plants and trees change their upward trajectory to pass between rocks or paving stones and preserve their strength. 'Bright and Clear' is a point on the Gallbladder meridian, the partner of the Liver official. It helps us to see our plan and decide whether or not it is still appropriate before we forge ahead. With these two points, I hoped that Ella would begin to let go of her vice-like grip on everything and allow her life to unfold in a more fluid and natural way.

* * *

Two weeks later, a surprisingly demure version of Ella arrived. Her hair was hanging loose and she seemed more at ease with herself. She even asked me about my weekend. I was surprised and intrigued by her warmth. It was yet more evidence that the treatments were really starting to deliver. Once the pleasantries were over, she leaned forward and rested her elbows on her knees.

"Do you want to hear something strange?"

"Be my guest."

"I had lunch with Carl last week. There was a really good-looking man sitting in the corner of the restaurant on his own and I kept on catching his eye. Carl actually turned around to see who I was looking at, which was a bit embarrassing. Anyway, I went home and that was that, but then the next morning I took the Eurostar to Paris and there he was again, in the queue. He clocked me and we smiled at each other."

"Amazing! Did you speak to him?"

"No, I didn't, and I was kicking myself for the rest of the journey. I even took my laptop to the restaurant carriage, hoping that he might wander in for a coffee. I felt like a stalker! I am *not* someone who chases men. But wait, it gets even weirder. That evening, I went out for dinner and I saw him again! He was with someone and I was with a client, so there was nothing I could do, but we locked eyes and he smiled at me as he left the restaurant. What are the chances of that?"

Ella's tale of serendipity was intriguing but the most remarkable thing for me was not so much the story as the storyteller. The way she spoke was the sound of springtime, full of hope, possibility and the unexpected. It was a far cry from the bossy, humourless woman I had met a few weeks earlier. Still, rather than get caught up in the drama, I dared to suggest that maybe her mystery man was just a messenger, the fleeting avatar of a new-found ability to see outside of the cage in which she had imprisoned herself. Her nod of approval told me that my suggestion had struck a chord. Whether or not the handsome stranger showed up in her life again, the very fact that something outside of her plan had made her feel this way seemed to be causing her to consider the possibility that it could happen again.

The Liver official governs vision and perception,

enabling us to make plans based on what we see not only with the physical eye but also with the mind and the spirit. Each of the five elements has its own spirit or nature. In the case of the Wood element, it is the Three Hun, which rule over the domain of dreams, fantasy and imagination. It is said that when we die, the Three Hun rise and return to heaven, while their counterpart, the Seven Po – associated with the Metal element – remain on earth. It is this separation that we call "death". The Liver official knows that everything is possible, that there are no limitations, and that the ultimate freedom is the freedom not to be free.

On the upper part of our back is an acupuncture point called 'Soul Door'. It is here that spirit enters and becomes our unique soul. Further down the same meridian, we find 'Spiritual Soul Gate', the place where the Three Hun come and go. It is said that at eleven o'clock each night, they become restless and leave our physical body to travel freely in time and space. This is what we experience as the dream state. Unhindered by the limitations of the body and the conscious mind, the Three Hun enable us to expand our consciousness, reflecting on what we already know about ourselves and also, importantly, giving us glimpses of what we can become. At three o'clock in the morning, they return to the body, entering through the same gate from which they left. In the West, we analyse dreams in an attempt to understand what they symbolise and therefore what they tell us about the psyche. In this tradition, however, the dream state demonstrates our capacity to experience unlimited freedom, something that we don't enjoy in our normal conscious existence.

* * *

By the time Ella came back for her next appointment, summer was in full swing. Her menstrual cycle had reset itself, shifting from the full moon to the new moon, and for the first time in her life she had no pain. What is more, the flow of blood had reduced to three days. She seemed pleased, but as soon as I asked her how she had been since our last session, her mood changed. She told me that she hadn't been able to get the mystery man off her mind. After agonising over it for a week or so, she had gone back to the restaurant where she had first seen him and asked the manager if she would mind giving him a letter.

"What made you think he would go back there?"

"It was obvious that he was a regular. I could tell from the way he interacted with the staff. The manager knew exactly who I was referring to when I described him. She told me she would be happy to give him the letter."

"What did you write to him?"

"I just said that it seemed so serendipitous that our paths had crossed so many times. I gave him my number and asked him to get in touch if he would like to meet up."

"Well done! That's great, Ella."

"Yes, except for one thing. He sent me a text message yesterday to say that he couldn't meet up."

"Did he give a reason?"

"Yes. He's married."

Ella was crestfallen but I was impressed that she had taken such a bold step. "Good for you for taking a risk. I would have done the same."

It felt like a poignant moment but Ella wasn't in the mood for reflection. She slapped her knees and looked me squarely in the eyes. "I'm going to go it alone."

"I'm sorry?"

"I've decided to find a sperm donor. I'm going to need your help."

My line of work never fails to amaze me. Had I been asked to guess what Ella would do next it would not have been this, yet now that she had said it, it seemed so obvious. She was approaching forty, she was very comfortably off and she was probably the most proactive and organised person I had ever met. She also had two ex-partners who were completely devoted to her. If anyone could make a success of this, it was her. She was a changed woman. She had become easy company, albeit still a touch bossy, and she was fully invested in the treatment process. I recommended a local clinic that could help with the *in vitro* fertilisation aspect of the process and an agency in the USA that offered a large selection of sperm donors. She already had a clear picture in her mind of the donor she would like: tall, black, athletic and 'hot'. It felt like we were in totally new territory.

Ella needed no encouragement to get started with the treatment that day. She made her way enthusiastically over to the treatment couch and lay down with her palms facing upwards. "Let's do this!" she said. I was keen not to disturb the equilibrium that was now apparent both in her demeanour and her pulses. Now was the time to support the status quo and ensure that the changes I was witnessing were given every chance to take hold. I chose the 'associated effect points', which give the Liver and Gallbladder officials an encouraging lift. As the needle connected with the first point, Ella seemed to melt into the couch.

"Good job, Gerad. That hit the mark."

* * *

Ella's new plan was unveiled with great excitement and panache. She had created a slideshow which mapped out her fertility campaign in minute detail. Clinics had been listed with scores based on extensive research. Sperm donors had been placed into different categories and rated on a scale of one to five. There was a timeline that included exact dates for the IVF process, embryo testing, embryo transfer, birth, interviews with maternity nurses, elective caesarean, as well as every detail of how her work schedule would fit around all of this. The level of detail was both fascinating and migraine-inducing, but the part that really caught my attention was the list of guests to the baby shower. First and second on the list were Carl and Hakeem.

"Have you told them what you're planning?"

"Not yet. Once everything is in place, I'll run them through it and explain how they're going to fit in."

"Fit in?"

"They're going to be joint godfathers."

Old habits die hard. Ella was still in full planning mode, plotting her campaign like a general on the battlefield, but she was visibly more relaxed and energised. It felt like she was returning to form, free of the frustration of not being able to move forward in the way that she wanted. However, in the weeks that followed, she became increasingly headstrong and impatient. Contrary to my advice, she chose an IVF clinic that I was not familiar with, and despite her exhaustive research, she chose the very first donor that ticked all the boxes. I started to notice that her overall strategy was full of confusions and contradictions. I did my best to steer her through the process but most of my guidance or suggestions fell on deaf ears. I was beginning to see more clearly why her original plan hadn't materialised.

"Ella, I highly recommend that you get the embryos tested before transferring them."

"Why?"

"Because at your age there is a high chance of miscarriage. It's best to know that the embryo is viable or you could end up losing three months."

"Look, I'm fit and healthy and thanks to you my cycle is perfect. If I don't get on with it, I'm going to lose three months anyway. I'm doing what's right."

"Ella, whatever you decide to do, I will support you. Just bear in mind that I've been working in this field for a long time, so you might want to have a think about my advice."

Whenever I dared to question her plan, the reaction was instant. She would scrunch up her face and turn away in a vain attempt to hide her obvious displeasure. Then, a moment later, her head would snap back into place like an elastic band.

"I'm grateful for your opinion but I'm going to stick to my plan. The clinic told me that testing is a waste of money."

It was obvious that Ella only wanted to listen to people who told her what she wanted to hear. It was equally obvious that she was cross with me for having dared challenge her strategy. Apparently, her new project was reactivating the belligerent, intransigent woman I had first met and my fear was that her behaviour would alienate the very people on whom she was relying to help her realise her plan. Nevertheless, I felt that I had done all that I could to advise her in my role as a fertility expert. Now it was time to focus my attention on bringing her Wood officials back in line.

'Yang Mound Spring' is the perfect expression of how we feel when we are in our youth. 'Yang' evokes the feeling of something new. 'Mound' refers to the burial ground of the elders, whose wisdom guides us back to the path when we go astray. 'Spring' symbolises the vitality and optimism that enables us to engage fully with the present moment and embrace the future. The location of this point – just below the outer side of the knee – is significant. It gives us the strength to leap to our feet and seize the day, the flexibility to take calculated risks and expand our horizons, and the momentum to continually enjoy the limitless freedom that we have been given. I asked Ella to bend her knee, but just as I was preparing to needle the point, she straightened both her legs and folded her arms to indicate that she was no longer cooperating. I stopped what I was doing and sat down on the stool beside the treatment couch.

"Ella?"

"Why aren't you doing more points below my belly button?"

While she was constructing her new plan, Ella had done some research into so-called 'fertility acupuncture' and had become aware of certain protocols that would supposedly help her to get pregnant. She had compiled a list of points that she wanted me to use and on which days of the cycle I should use them. I had already explained that the practices she had read about were from a different acupuncture tradition and that I was not prepared to be given direction but it hadn't gone down well. Nevertheless, I had no intention of allowing myself to be coerced into doing something that was contrary to my way of working.

"Ella, I am very happy to help you through this process but as I explained to you before, the way I practise does not align with other acupuncture traditions. The points I choose are the ones that I think will be most beneficial to you. Where they are on the body is immaterial." She remained silent for the rest of the treatment but her body language was loud and clear. The rapport had been broken and unless I could re-establish it, the work with the needles would almost certainly not be as effective. "I understand how important this is for you. If you would prefer to see someone else, I can refer you to a good practitioner that uses the protocols you have cited."

She climbed down from the treatment couch without saying a word and got dressed. Before leaving the room, she turned to face me. "My PA will be in touch to schedule the next appointment. In the meantime, I'm going to reflect on what you have said." Ella left the room without saying goodbye. The following morning I received a short but polite email from her PA saying that she didn't want to make any more appointments at this time. It was another six months before I heard from her again.

* * *

As my mother was nearing the end of her life, I was sitting by her bedside one day when she suddenly opened her eyes and looked at me with a furrowed brow. "I've just realised that I've only lived through eighty-two springtimes," she said, before lapsing back into the morphine haze from which she had emerged.

Her words made me panic. "That's not a lot," I thought. "I wonder how many I have left?" I looked at the fresh green shoots sprouting from the sapling outside her window and all of a sudden I felt the most enormous sense of gratitude that Nature was giving me yet another chance to express this precious gift of life, another chance to grow. As I sat by my mother's side, I was filled with sadness that her life was coming to an end, but in that moment, I resolved once more to make the most of my own, to live it to the fullest no matter what might stand in my way.

This powerful feeling of determination and hope for

the future is precisely what the Wood element and its associated season, the spring, gives us. As my mother gently folded her wings and surrendered to death, the young tree outside her window stretched its arms towards the heavens. One life was ending and another was beginning in this never-ending cycle of existence.

When Ella eventually reappeared at my clinic, she looked battle weary. It was a year since she had first come to see me and spring was once again in the air, but her energy was definitely not in sync with the season. She lifted herself laboriously out of the chair in the waiting room and gave herself a good stretch. I told her how pleased I was to see her again and she returned the compliment, but the look of defeat in her eyes betrayed what she was feeling. She told me that not long after our last session together, the sperm had arrived from the States and the IVF process had kicked off in earnest. Ten eggs had been collected, four of them had been fertilised and two of them had survived to day six. One had been frozen, while the other had been transferred for implantation purposes. Ten days later, the pregnancy test came back negative. She was advised to do another round and an almost identical pattern emerged. Again, she was advised to keep going, but this time the cycle was abandoned due to low follicular development. She then transferred the two frozen embryos, but again the pregnancy test came back negative. She was physically and emotionally exhausted.

"I'm done, I can't do this any more. You have no idea what it's like. Endless sheets of paper telling me when to inject this, when to take that, scans at seven in the morning, people poking and prodding you. Week after week I've been haemorrhaging money and for what? It's all been a complete waste of time." Even though I could still sense the underlying fury and frustration, losing the battle had clearly drained her.

"How best can I help you at this point, Ella?"

"I just want to get myself back. I don't know who I am any more."

"Who's been supporting you through all of this?"

"No one. Nobody knows." I was a little surprised that she hadn't confided in her two ex-partners. Then again, she may have been loath to tip the balance of power by showing her vulnerability. When I haven't seen a patient for over three months, I try to start again with a clean slate. It's always useful to reassess the original diagnosis and often you see and sense things that you missed the first time around. I was still happy with my diagnosis of the Wood element as the Causative Factor, but there was a certain humility and vulnerability that I hadn't noticed before. I had the sense that she had finally placed her trust in me rather than seeing what I could offer her as one small part of a larger plan. In order to work out a treatment strategy, I needed to ask myself some simple questions. What was it about the Liver and Gallbladder officials that was disturbing the overall balance? What was it that Ella really wanted? And how would I gauge if we were successful? I decided to jot down some notes:

1. Liver creating well-formed but rigid plans. No room to evolve.
2. Gallbladder unable to cope with inflexibility and lack of communication.
3. Wants normal life with loving partner, friends and family.

When they are in balance, the Wood Officials complement each other perfectly and the process of creation unfolds effortlessly. The Liver Official, known as the general of the armed forces, comes up with the strategy. The Gallbladder Official, representing the foot soldiers, puts the plan into action but lets the general know if the strategy isn't working. In Ella's case, the plan had been non-negotiable, so the Gallbladder official had not even been consulted. My aim was to select points that would strengthen the Liver and Gallbladder officials equally so that neither of them would feel more or less important. In the Huangdi Neijing, the Liver and Gallbladder officials are described as being as close as a "hand in a glove", emphasising the importance of absolute synergy between the two of them.

Ella came weekly for treatment with the simple desire to feel well and, in stark contrast to our earlier sessions, was conciliatory and compliant. There was a sense of surrender, an acknowledgement that she could no longer rely on self will alone. My treatment room became a space for her to practise being vulnerable, to express her fears and her failings. I enjoyed witnessing her transformation and always looked forward to our sparring, which by now had become playful rather than antagonistic. Slowly but surely, she started to find her feet again and one by one the changes began to bubble to the surface.

"You know what? I feel like a teenager again. When I was growing up in Berlin, I was free as a bird and full of confidence, despite the fact that I stuck out like a sore thumb. The area we lived in was very white but I didn't care. I liked being different."

"What changed?"

"The onset of puberty, I guess. I suddenly became very self-conscious and my whole outlook changed. I was angry."

"About what?"

"The injustice of it all. I was angry that my parents hadn't prepared us properly for life in the West. I was angry that my uniqueness was perceived to be an obstacle. Everywhere I looked I saw oppression and it was always people like me that bore the brunt. I just wanted to run. That's why I applied to study in London. In the end, my anger was my saviour."

I couldn't help but admire Ella's fierce and courageous spirit. Dislocation and difference had defined her childhood and followed her as she struck out on her own in a new country, but although the memory of her childhood was troubling, the way in which she described it to me had no charge to it. The atmosphere in the room was uplifting and she seemed full of optimism. Was this the real Ella?

* * *

The following week, Ella was transformed. When I walked into the waiting room to collect her, she leapt to her feet and announced with great excitement that she had something to tell me. Unconsciously, I found myself responding to her energy and skipped down the stairs in a fashion most unlike me. She sauntered into the treatment room and threw her jacket onto the back of the armchair with a flourish.

"You seem very bright and breezy, Ella."

"Bright and breezy doesn't even begin to describe the way I feel!"

"Wonderful! That's music to my ears. Tell me what's been happening."

"Making amends, that's what's been happening. I've been reading some self-help books and one of the recurrent themes is making amends to people you've wronged."

"Step Nine."

"Step what?"

"Making amends to people is Step Nine in the Twelve Step programme."

"I'll take your word for it. Anyway, I decided to do it myself."

"That's wonderful, Ella. Maybe you should start with me?"

"Very funny. Seriously, though, I thought long and hard about the people I've wronged in the past and it was a sobering experience. I'm not ready to start making amends to everyone, but there was one person I felt compelled to apologise to right away and that was Hakeem. I was so tough on him, you know? God knows why he's stood by me all this time. I took him out to dinner last week and apologised for the way I had treated him."

"That's impressive, Ella. It's not an easy thing to do."

Ella slipped her shoes off and pulled her legs up onto the chair as she always did when she was about to share something important. "I admitted that I had blamed him for the failure of the IVF without any justification. I told him that I had let him go because he didn't fit into my plan any more. I remember thinking it was the only logical thing to do at the time but in retrospect it seemed so brutal. It felt good to be honest about it."

"I'm happy for you, Ella. What you did takes a lot of courage and I'm sure Hakeem will have appreciated it."

"He was so sweet and forgiving. We talked for hours and hours and I felt like I was getting to know him in a way that I hadn't before. I was so blinkered when we were together. It was all about getting what I wanted. At the end of the evening, he started crying and told me that he had never stopped loving me. Then he asked me if I would consider giving it another go."

"So… what did you say?"

"I said yes!" Ella burst into tears and then almost immediately started laughing. "You see what you've done to me? I never cry!"

In the ancient Chinese tradition, there is a natural hierarchy to which the officials belong. The ruler of the kingdom is the Heart official, the supreme controller. Second in line is the Lung official, who acts as the prime minister. Beneath them is the Liver official, the general of the armed forces. When the instruments of power cooperate, authority, diplomacy and the peaceful expansion of the kingdom are the natural outcomes. Everyone knows their role and everything they do is for the common good. When one or other of the officials falls out of line, however, that natural symbiotic harmony is lost and the resulting chaos is inevitable. In Ella's case, the Liver official had failed to offer a coherent plan for growth and renewal. Without it, the Heart and Lung officials had struggled to provide the leadership that the other officials needed to function as they should. Now, finally, with the Liver official performing its rightful duties, the Heart official was back in control and the natural order was restored.

10

VERY GREAT ABYSS

*

One morning in early October, I was preparing my treatment room for the day ahead when Eszter came downstairs to tell me that my first patient of the day had cancelled. Taking advantage of the opportunity to run some errands, I put on my coat and headed out into the street. It was one of those bright, crisp autumn mornings when the sun is low in the sky and everything is bathed in an amber glow. I switched on my phone and it immediately beeped at me. It was a voice message from my dog walker, Jennifer. She told me that her best friend had just come out of hospital after an acute attack of diverticulitis and was very weak and distressed. She asked if I could fit him in for an urgent appointment. I hesitated for a moment. Half of me wanted to say no, but the better angels of my nature reminded me that most of my errands could wait, so I messaged her back to say that I could see him at nine. When I returned to the clinic half an hour later, I saw an elderly man emerging from a cab and climbing the steps that led to the front door. As he reached the top, a gust of wind dislodged his hat, sending it spinning into the gutter. I stooped to pick it up, ran up the steps and handed it to him.

"Let me get the door for you." The man brushed me aside with a dismissive gesture, screwed up his face and began peering at the names on the buzzers. "If you'll allow me, I have the keys."

"Go on, then. What are you waiting for?" I turned the key in the lock, swung open the door and ushered him in with an exaggerated gesture of welcome that I regretted as soon as I had made it. It is in moments such as this that I am reminded of the two distinctly different hats that I wear in life. There's the personal 'me' that reacts to the behaviour of others and then there's the professional 'me' that observes it with nothing but curiosity in order to make a diagnosis. In this awkward encounter, the professional 'me' had been absent. Still somewhat flustered, I headed down to my treatment room to get everything ready. A few minutes later, Eszter appeared in the doorway clutching an armful of toilet rolls.

"What's up, Eszter?" She pinched her nose with her thumb and forefinger.

"I'm fine. I just wish people would do their business before they leave home. You're alright down here but I'm right in the firing line. Anyway, your patient is upstairs."

"OK, I'll be up in a minute. Who is it? Please don't tell me it's that man I just let into the building…"

"Yes, it is. His name is John."

I felt a rush of shame. "I should have guessed. Eszter, he's come straight from the hospital. Would you ask him if he needs anything?" Before I was conscious of what I was doing, I started running a finger over the surfaces to check for dust, before running upstairs to the waiting room. In the far corner, I saw a bedraggled figure brushing the dirt from his hat.

"Good morning, sir!" No response. I walked over to his chair and held out my hand to greet him. "We meet again! I'm Gerad." He tipped his hat onto the floor beside his chair, grabbed my hand with both of his and lifted himself to his feet with a loud grunt.

"John. Jennifer's friend." The soulless look that met my eyes took me by surprise.

"Pleased to meet you, John. My room is this way." I gestured towards the door but he didn't move. Instead, he mumbled something and pointed towards the floor. For the second time that morning, I bent down to retrieve his hat. Beneath it were a pair of leather gloves and a cotton shoulder bag, out of which an old book with frayed edges had spilled.

"Theosophy."

"I'm sorry?"

"The book. It's on theosophy."

"I see."

"These beautiful old buildings have been wrecked," he announced, wagging his finger at the circular metal light hanging from the ornate ceiling rose above him. "Look at it! It's a monstrosity." I invited him to follow me, but when we reached the staircase he stopped and stared with undisguised disgust at the newly laminated floor, which he tapped with the toe of his shoe.

"Ugh!"

"Follow me, John. I'll walk in front of you. If you fall, you can fall on me. My grandmother taught me that."

"I should think so."

I love my treatment room. It's a bright and airy space with simple but elegant furniture and windows that give onto the courtyard garden above. Most of my patients love it too, and often comment on how peaceful it feels. When John entered the room, he said nothing and seemed to be either unaware of, or uninterested in, his new surroundings.

"Take a seat, John. I'll get you some water."

"You've got a cracked pane up there," he said, pointing to one of the skylights as he lowered himself into the armchair. I nodded and handed him a glass of water before taking my seat. John was in his early eighties but his hollow eyes and unkempt appearance made him look older. He wore elegant but rather dirty clothes that had long since lost their shape and smelled of an old, musty wardrobe. His face was sallow with blotches of eczema and patches of stubble that he had missed when shaving. Crowning his head was a shapeless mop of thinning white hair that he had tucked behind his ears. We sat in silence for a few moments and then, all of a sudden, his hand shot upwards like the tongue of a lizard to catch a moth that had been circling his head. "They'll eat everything, you know. You'll have to strip the entire building and start again." He opened his fist, tipped the lifeless moth onto the floor and blew the dust from the palm of his hand. I watched him, fascinated by the spectacle, and waited for him to settle.

"It's good to meet you, John. I'm sorry to hear that you've been unwell. I understand you've been in hospital."

"It was hellish. Non-stop noise and that infuriating beeping sound all night long. I discharged myself early this morning and called Jennifer. She said I should see you and I thought, well, I've got nothing else to do today, so here I am." For a split second I felt hurt by his comment but I quickly gathered myself and swallowed my pride. Nevertheless, I felt conflicted. Here was an elderly man who had just endured a sleepless night in hospital, yet I felt no sympathy for him. I sat forward in my chair and smiled at him but, just as I was about to ask my next question, he placed one hand on his stomach and let out a long, hissing belch from the corner of his mouth. He seemed unaware that it might cause offence. To such an extent, in fact, that he immediately let out an even louder one without any attempt to disguise it. I sat back, feeling somewhat defeated.

"I understand from Jennifer that you've had a nasty bout of diverticulitis. Inflammation of the large intestine, right? Can you give me a bit of the history? How long have you had it for?"

"Oh, I don't know. Most of my friends are dropping like flies. I hope I won't be the last one standing."

"It must be hard getting older and seeing your friends suffer."

"And if you value your carpet, you'll do something about these moths right now. Their eggs will already be gestating in the weave, waiting to hatch." I persevered with my questioning for a while but it felt laboured and fruitless. However hard I tried, he seemed reluctant to divulge any of his symptoms or his medical history, let alone anything about himself. By the end of the consultation, I had half a page of scribbled notes and no real sense of the man sitting in front of me. I had no choice but to work with what I had.

"OK, I've got enough for the first treatment, John. I'm going to wash my hands quickly. Would you care to lie on the treatment couch?"

He threw his arms into the air. "Do I have a choice?"

* * *

John was not easy to get on with. My gestures of warmth and my willingness to listen felt wasted on him; yet, despite his hostility, the blank look in his eyes triggered a desire within me to pull him from the void in which he seemed to be trapped. I also suspected that he had something to teach me. The people we find most difficult are often the ones from whom we learn the most, just as the most challenging situations often end up being the most rewarding. I could simply have written him off as a grouchy and unpleasant old man, but that would have been to misunderstand the root cause of his behaviour and miss the way in which he was telling me – without words – how much he was struggling. I had yet to make a diagnosis, but the brusque encounter on the clinic steps, his inability to engage in a respectful and meaningful way, and his apparent reluctance to provide the information I needed, reminded me of the way it feels to be in the presence of someone who is grieving. It seems as though they are rejecting the outside world, but in fact they just need space to come to terms with the weight of their loss. This jarring sense of bereavement suggested to me that the root of his imbalance might well be the Metal element, the associated emotion of which is grief.

Witnessing my mother's death taught me a lot about grief. Her final hours were painful and distressing, and the morphine did little to ease her discomfort. The experience of holding her hand at the moment of death touched me deeply and gave me a visceral appreciation of the most dramatic contrast of all: that between the fullness of life and the empty, neutralised state of death. As she gripped my hand with every ounce of her remaining strength, I was engulfed by everything she ever was, and then she was gone. As I sat beside her lifeless body, I felt as if I were staring into the abyss, an eternal void without form or memory.

One of the fundamental principles of Taoist philosophy is the concept of oneness. It is this overarching connectivity that gives us a sense of our rightful place in the universe. Importantly, it also gives us the ability to connect with ourselves and others, both in the present moment and through memory. This natural capacity is governed by the Metal element and all of its many manifestations. In ancient times, precious metals and gems were believed to connect us to our spiritual roots, as well as being potent symbols of rank, identity and status. Nowadays, we value metals primarily for their role in creating the technology that enables us to connect with each other across vast distances. Whether or not we realise it, everyone and everything is connected by the power of the Metal element, both within and without. Most of us take this reassuring and grounding experience for granted until something as simple as becoming disconnected from the internet happens. All of a sudden we feel lost and alone. For people who have an imbalance in the Metal element, this feeling is a daily reality.

To understand the nature of Metal, we need to pay attention to the season of autumn and what it teaches us. Autumn is the dying season, the time when Nature strips away the old to make space for the new. In the human body, the Metal element is represented by the Lung official and the Large Intestine official. The lungs receive oxygen, or the "pure qi from the heavens", as it is referred to in the Taoist classics, while the Large Intestine official is responsible for the identification and removal of waste. With every in-breath and out-breath, the Metal element perfectly balances the new and the old, silently managing the space within us and keeping us connected to all that is above and below. It gives us our rightful place in life as we stand between Father Heaven and Mother Earth.

The treatment I had given John that first day was simple and, as ever, Nature had shown me what to do. The colour in his face was ghostly white and his voice had a soft, weeping quality, as if he were mourning a loss. His odour was rotten, like someone or something in the early stages of decomposition. And the predominant emotion was grief, a profound aura of emptiness and bereavement.

VERY GREAT ABYSS

These four pieces of sensory phenomena, all produced by the Metal element as a distress call from within, directed me to two points on the Lung and Large Intestine meridians. As I needled the last of the two points, John let out a satisfied sigh. I took his hand to read his pulse again and then held it for a little while longer to witness the change in him. At the beginning of the session, his hands had felt cold and moist. Now there was a warming and softening that radiated through me.

"Are we done?" he asked.

"Yes, we're done. The first treatment is short and sweet but pay attention to how you feel from now on. Your feedback will help me to know if I am on the right track." He raised his eyebrows and looked at me doubtfully.

"If you say so."

* * *

When John returned the following week, I was surprised. In fact, I was so sure that he wouldn't come back that I had already put on my coat to go out when the buzzer sounded. My heart sank, and this unusual reaction took me by surprise. Why was I not excited to discover how my patient had responded to the first treatment? Had I given up on him already? Had his negativity rubbed off on me? I took off my coat, reset myself and headed up to the waiting room where I found John standing in the middle of the reception area, holding court.

"I went to the same drama school as all the greats, you know. Gielgud, Attenborough, Olivier. The list goes on.

I would have acted in the movies but I couldn't bear the thought of living in Los Angeles, so I stuck to television. I had plenty of offers, mind you. I turned down several films that ended up going to lesser actors."

Eszter was wide-eyed with excitement. "Gerad! John knows Hugh Grant. Oh, and he was in that TV ad. You know, the one with the little girl and her grandfather."

I noticed a flash of irritation as John stepped towards me with his hand outstretched. "That's not *all* I've done. I do commercials to pay the bills between serious acting jobs." I was struck by how different he looked compared to the first time we had met. He was dressed in a smart fawn suit with a red handkerchief poking out of the top pocket and his skin was glistening. It was a reassuring sight. I led him downstairs, excited to hear how he had been since the last treatment.

"How are you doing, John?"

"I'm OK."

"Have you noticed any changes since we last met? You look much better."

"My gut feels a little better. It's probably all that water you told me to drink."

"Better? How much better."

"A bit better."

"On a scale of one to ten?" He scrunched up his face and looked at me as if I had just said something stupid. "Let's say you were a two last week. How much better are you today?"

"I don't know. Seven?"

"Quite a lot better then."

"If you say so."

His continual unwillingness to engage in an open and productive way was tiresome and difficult. There is always a part of me that wants a patient to wax lyrical about how much better they feel, but this was different. His demeanour not only felt obstructive but completely bereft of warmth.

"Have you noticed any other changes this past week? Maybe in how you feel in yourself or how you have felt around other people?" John said nothing. Every attempt I made to further our relationship and collect information was met with a blank stare. From my clinical perspective, John was neither difficult nor obstructive. It was simply that he was incapable of taking anything in. I knew that if I wanted to find a way to connect with him and give him the help he needed, I would need to be sensitive and respectful, just as you would with someone in the early stages of grief. "John, I get the sense that you have lived an interesting life. It would be really helpful to hear more about you and your past. Would that be OK?" I spoke slowly and carefully as I ventured into his misty world. "Perhaps you could tell me about a time in your life when you felt content and fulfilled?"

He seemed surprised by the change of direction and remained still for a few moments, glancing at me occasionally as if to check that the delay in responding was acceptable. Finally, just as I was about to move on to another question, he began talking.

"The only time in my life when I really felt a part of something was when I was on the Hippie Trail in the early sixties. It was a time when many of us were searching for authentic experiences, and the East became a kind of mecca. I was in my early thirties and although I was finding plenty of work as an actor, I hadn't achieved the recognition I thought I was worthy of. I guess I was looking for something else to give my life some meaning. I thought I would find it on the Trail."

He sat back in the chair, lost in thought, and stared at the skylight. The change of atmosphere in the room was palpable. When he returned his gaze to me, there seemed to be a flicker of light emerging from the abyss. "I bought myself an old VW camper van and drove it across the Alps to northern Italy. From there I drove to Sarajevo and then down through the Balkans to northern Greece and Turkey." As he spoke, his face lit up and his body softened. "I will never forget arriving in Istanbul. The sights, the sounds, the smells, the call to prayer. It all felt so alien and yet it was intensely alluring. For the first time in my life I felt as if I were entering into a mystery with no idea of what might happen. It was magical."

The sudden transformation from empty shell to inspired storyteller threw me in the most delightful way. It was like being in the room with a totally different person. And the way that he spoke was fascinating. Rather than describing the usual excitements of a road trip adventure, he created an atmosphere that was poignant and profound. I was captivated. "After Istanbul, I drove all the way across the Middle East as far as Kabul. From there I crossed the Khyber Pass into Pakistan and then on to India. My final destination was Varanasi, the spiritual capital." As he spoke, the subtle movements of his face and eyes betrayed a time that was clearly of great importance to him.

"Can you still remember that feeling from Istanbul?"

"Oh yes. Like it was yesterday."

We sat for a moment in silence, the connection between us finally established. The warmth and trust that he exuded was so intimate and touching that I could scarcely believe this was the same man that had been so cold and dismissive on the day of our first encounter. It was clear to me that what John most needed was to reconnect with something inside himself. Something to elevate his mundane existence. Something beyond his logical mind, with all of its distracting and self-defeating ideas about the world and his place in it.

'Soul Door' is an acupuncture point located on the upper back, directly over the lungs. Its function is to receive 'spirit' and transform it into each individual's unique manifestation of that force. Our soul maintains our connection with our origin (the Tao) and helps us to find meaning in life, not from mental calculations of good and bad but from a permanent, peaceful state of being that is beyond such comparisons. I ended the second treatment with the 'tonification points', which enact the Law of Mother/Child. According to this law, each element creates and nourishes the following element in the cycle of creation, just as a mother gives birth to, and feeds, her child. On this occasion, the points I chose would draw energy from the Earth element (the mother) to the Metal element (her child).

THE UNTAPPED SELF

I escorted John back up to the reception area where Eszter was on all fours, picking up the post that had been pushed through the letterbox. As John approached, she stood up, opened the door and smiled at him. "Goodbye, Mr Bryant. I enjoyed talking to you earlier." John stepped outside and disappeared without saying a word. As the door closed behind him, a gust of wind blew inside, scattering the remaining letters across the floor. As I sat in the back of a cab heading home that evening, I stared out of the rain-splattered window and wondered how it was that John had disappeared into his untouchable space again so quickly. When he left the clinic that day, Eszter had looked up and joined me in a profound feeling of sadness and disappointment. It was heavy and soul-sapping, and I couldn't help wondering if what we both felt in that moment was John's prevailing emotional state.

* * *

The following weekend, the autumn rain fell without a break, so I surrendered to the sofa and the comfort of my two dogs and the television. As I was flicking from one station to the next in search of something to watch, I suddenly came across a comedy series from the 1980s, in which John had a starring role. I was transfixed. How on earth could this bright star have become so tarnished? Had something terrible happened in his life, or had he somehow managed to compartmentalise the light and the shade within him? I started to do a bit of research and discovered that almost all of his characters made light of subject matter that was generally considered taboo. He was a master of dark humour.

In general, John was more cheerful than when he had first come to see me, but by now I knew that it was futile asking him to tell me how he felt. I would have to rely on my own observations. During our previous session, he had come alive when talking about his days on the Hippie Trail, so I tried to pick up where we had left off. I was anxious to know if the connection between us could be rekindled.

"I'd love to hear more about your journey to the East, John." He lifted his head and stared at me without a trace of emotion. And then, after a long period of silence, he reached across and placed his ghost-like fingers on my hand.

"Do you believe in God?" His question totally threw me, but my instinct told me that I should take my time before answering.

"I am aware of my own existence… Maybe that is what God means to me?" John slowly pulled his hand away, sat back in his chair and looked up towards the skylight. I felt like a child waiting to hear if I had passed a test. After what felt like an eternity, he lowered his eyes and smiled gently.

"Can I have the needles now?"

John changed our relationship that day. Despite his negativity and unwillingness to engage, I had the feeling that he trusted and respected me, but it had quickly become more than that. I had the sense that he had placed me on a pedestal, that he thought he could find what he was looking for in me. It was not the first time that I had experienced something like this. Sometimes, the intimacy and intensity of the therapeutic relationship is such that the patient begins to deify the practitioner. Thankfully, he decided to question if I was indeed the saviour and quickly discovered that I wasn't. Despite the polite smile, my answer to his question about my belief in God had provoked a brief but noticeable flash of disappointment. In the weeks that followed, I got the sense that he was committed to the treatment process but had understood that his search for the ultimate connection was one that he would have to undertake alone.

* * *

Despite his somewhat gloomy demeanour, I could see that John was making progress. The problems with his digestive system had cleared up, his health seemed to be better and despite his occasionally obstructive manner with me, I noticed that he was striking up a friendly rapport with Eszter. Generally speaking, when a patient is on the up and their symptoms have diminished but not yet disappeared, monthly maintenance sessions are enough to keep them in balance. When I suggested this to John, however, he baulked at the idea and insisted on coming every other week. Summer came and went and as October approached, I remembered that it would soon be a year since he first came to see me. The previous autumn had been wet and cold, but this year was different. The late summer warmth had given way to cool, clear days, and my treatment room was flooded with glorious autumnal sunlight when John arrived for his next appointment.

"Today's the day, John. It's exactly one year since you first came to see me. How are we going to celebrate our anniversary?" He sat still and said nothing. "Are you OK, John?"

"There's something I want you to know." He reached into his jacket pocket, pulled out a brown envelope and handed it to me. Inside was an old newspaper cutting with a head shot of John in his younger years. Above it was a headline that read: "Actor kills son in tragic accident."

"Do you want to talk about this, John?"

John shook his head slowly. "I just wanted you to know. That's enough."

* * *

The correlation between Taoist philosophy and modern science is striking. According to contemporary thinking, space did not exist prior to the Big Bang. Rather, it emerged from a single unmanifest entity in a cosmic explosion that expanded into billions of galaxies. For Taoists, the source of all life is the 'Tao', which is also beyond description or comprehension by the human mind. As it says in the Tao Te Ching, "The Tao that can be spoken of is not the eternal Tao." According to Taoist philosophy, space, the five elements and all of life emerged as a result of the opposing forces of yin and yang. Both theories highlight the significance of space and how it exists as the cause of everything we know. In Five-Element theory, it is the Metal element that governs space. It maintains our connection to every part of ourselves, our environment and the universe. Should the Metal element fail in its remit, our sense of belonging is broken and like the astronaut that has become separated from the spaceship, we feel alienated and alone, floating in space. 'Very Great Abyss' is the point on the Lung official meridian that re-establishes our connection with the source of our existence, just like the newborn child whose very first reflex is to fill its lungs with life-sustaining breath, kickstarting the process that will sustain it until the end of its life.

Learning about the death of John's son was surprising and shocking. How do you carry on living, knowing that you were responsible for your own child's death? How does anyone recover from that? If Nature has equipped us with all that we need to survive, what is it that enables us to recover from something as traumatic as this? Or are we doomed? It's not always easy to see when someone is healing. Like the iceberg that only shows a fraction of its total form, most of us reveal very little of ourselves on the surface. With many of my patients, the process of resolving past trauma and returning to balance happens imperceptibly. Sometimes they tell me when they are getting better. Sometimes there is no need because the way they present tells me everything I need to know. Occasionally, albeit rarely, I never find out. The Five-Element model of healing recognises that true healing can only happen once the cause of the imbalance has been addressed. Without that, any change in symptoms or inappropriate behaviour will only be temporary. The unexpected disclosure of this terrible tragedy suggested that the attachment to his past suffering was starting to give way to something new. For decades, he had been plagued by what he described as the living hell of guilt, fear and self-recrimination. Now, the possibility of redemption was beginning to seem like a possibility.

Nature teaches us about the cycles of life, including the process of death and rebirth. We are essentially a recycling unit for all of our experiences in life. Everything, good and bad alike, is processed and sorted. Anything that is beneficial to our health and wellbeing is retained. Everything else is excreted. It's not that we forget life's more challenging or painful events; it's that the emotional charge we produce in response to the event is naturally removed by the Metal. In John's case, his Metal failed to correctly evaluate his tragic loss, so rather than forgive himself and heal, he remained trapped in a state that felt like eternal damnation.

There are few points as powerful as 'Joining of the Valleys' (or 'The Great Eliminator', as it is commonly known) when it comes to helping someone release themselves from the scars of the past. This point, found on the meridian of the Large Intestine official, enables us to identify and remove anything that no longer has value or serves a purpose, be it toxic waste products, old resentments or a sense of guilt arising from wrongdoing. This process is also known as forgiveness, an innate capacity that enables us to cut ourselves free from the past and move on.

"Gerad, I want you to know that you've really helped

me over the past year. I have moments when the pain of my existence lessens and I get a brief glimpse of something other than failure and deep self-loathing." As was his wont, John sat back in his chair and looked up towards the heavens, lost in thought. The breeze had picked up a little, sweeping crimson-coloured leaves across the skylight and filling the room with that distinctive autumnal scent of decay. I joined him in silence, allowing him the time and space to reflect on what he had just told me, and then brought him gently back to the room.

"Do *you* believe in God, John?"

He closed his eyes, rubbed his face and turned his head slowly from side to side. "I do Gerad, yes. For a long time I lost my faith, but in recent months I've noticed myself marvelling at simple things again. After my son's death, I couldn't make sense of anything. Life seemed utterly pointless and even when I had moments of joy, I would punish myself and the people around me for feeling that way."

"What happened to your wife, John?"

"The accident tore us apart. She couldn't find it in herself to forgive me. She left me for one of my best friends. There was nothing I could do. I returned to London and took up acting again."

"I'm glad you did, John. You're a natural."

"It's a shame nobody else noticed."

* * *

Each time John came to see me, I was struck by how little

I had written in his file. My notes would typically read 'OK' or 'Better' or 'More gas'. But I was also struck by how little I knew about him personally. Usually my patients are willing, even eager, to tell me about the ups and downs of their lives. With John, it was different. It had been clear from the start that he wasn't inclined to say much about himself, so apart from my initial attempts to make a connection, I rarely ventured there. When I did, his tendency was to dismiss or ignore my questions as if they were pointless and irrelevant. Maybe he was right. Who wants to be asked about the mundane details of life when all you want is the space and silence to connect with something more important? In short, I realised that his story was not the story.

If I wanted to maintain any kind of rapport with him, I first had to understand that he never meant to be rude or dismissive. As off-putting as it was, that was just his way. If I then made the effort to penetrate the mist that enveloped him, I discovered a warmth and gravitas that I rarely found in others. When I think back to the time that we spent together over the years, I realise that much of it was in silence. I would begin by asking him something, and he would look me in the eyes without a flicker of emotion, drawing me into the void just as my mother had done when she was dying. It was as if he were waiting for me to remember that the key to his soul would only be found through profound connection.

John's response to acupuncture treatment was mixed. He told me that he felt a significant boost in his emotional and physical health for the first week after each treatment, but by the time he came back to see me at the end of the fortnight, he was generally withdrawn, struggling to sleep and experiencing recurrent bouts of abdominal pain. My interventions seemed to be maintaining him in the short term, but clearly there was something preventing him from returning to full health. Eighteen months into treatment, John collapsed while climbing up onto the treatment couch. Had I not been there to catch him, he would have fallen backwards onto the floor. I helped him settle but his breathing was laboured and irregular. Then, when I took his pulses, I noticed something new. The pulses on his left side were barely perceptible. I felt as if I were holding the hand of a dying man. I moved around the couch and picked up his right hand. The pulses were pumping hard and had a frenetic quality. There was only one thing this could mean.

Chinese medicine is based primarily on an understanding of the nature and movement of energy (qi). The rhythm and quality of energy as it moves around the body, mind and spirit mirrors the cycles that we see in Nature. For example, the pulses on the left wrist are collectively considered to be more yang (active). The energy of these pulses reflects the rising power of their associated seasons: winter, spring and summer. There is a real sense of life emerging from deep within, with all the power and promise of a new cycle. The pulses on the right wrist are collectively considered to be more yin (receptive). The energy of these pulses reflects the downward part of the cycle that we see in the late summer, autumn and winter as Nature slowly withdraws, lays down whatever she no longer needs and prepares for the next cycle. It is a perfectly balanced cycle of creation and destruction that ensures the continuity of life.

When the pulses on the left side resign, the pulses on the right respond to the emergency by going into overdrive, but there is only so long that such a desperate measure can be sustained. I took John's pulses a second time to be absolutely sure of what I was feeling. The readings were identical. John's energetic system was in a state of extreme imbalance and a separation of yin and yang would soon occur. This pattern indicated the beginning of organ failure, which would inevitably be followed by death. We have a treatment protocol that can in some cases restore the natural balance of the two sides, but in John's case it made no difference. No matter what I did, the pulses didn't change. I suggested that he see his doctor, and the following week he went back into hospital for further tests. The results were devastating. John had Stage Four cancer in the liver and bowel and was given three to six months to live. He decided against having chemotherapy, preferring to let Nature take her course. When I asked him how he felt about the diagnosis, he was calm and philosophical.

"I'm 83 years old, Gerad. I've had a good life but I'm tired. It's time to move on. I'd still like to come for treatment as long as I'm able to, though. Would that be OK?"

"Of course. I will do whatever I can to help you through this."

"I really wanted to go to Africa, you know. To see the animals."

"There's still time for that, John."

"Why didn't I do that? I'm so stupid." The weight of regret was heavy during our sessions. I tried to remind him of the good times, of his achievements, of his contribution to the world, but all of it fell on deaf ears. It seemed that he needed to lean on his misery to justify this sad, lonely and damning conclusion to his life.

John hadn't spoken about his son again, but I felt I should raise the subject one more time as he neared the end of his own life. I thought perhaps it would be cathartic. I thought about my time working on the AIDS ward in the early nineties and the ways in which the young people I was treating dealt with the knowledge of their imminent and untimely death. Many of them were profoundly distressed, angry and intensely lonely in their final days, yet there were some who, despite the tragedy of their situation and the stigma that hung over the ward, were able to accept their fate and find peace as death approached. One day, I plucked up the courage to ask him, treading carefully as I was unsure of how he would react.

"John, I've thought a great deal about your son's death and how profoundly it must have affected you. Have you been able to find peace with it?"

"I've lived a very interesting life, Gerad. I know it must seem like I only see the dark side but it's not the whole story by any means. Yes, I have found peace with the past and I have you to thank for that." He leaned forward and brushed my cheek with his hand. "The past can't hurt me any more." I will never forget that moment. The delicate gesture of affection and gratitude reminded me that the relationship between the patient and the practitioner is sacred. Words cannot express the bond. In the Huangdi Neijing, the bible of Five-Element Acupuncture, the work of the acupuncturist is described thus: "Healing is not nursing or mothering. The way to care for a patient is just to be yourself and be with him, looking into his eyes."

There's a poignancy to autumn. For all of its magnificent beauty, it is suffused with melancholy because it is a time of letting go. And yet there is also an air of anticipation, excitement even, for it is in letting go that something new is able to emerge. Therein lies the grace and majesty of the Metal element. John's peaceful acceptance of death was inspiring and reassuring, for despite his many regrets, I saw a frisson of excitement in his eyes when he wondered what lay beyond the veil. In the last two weeks of his life, he continued to visit me weekly, and I understood why regular treatments were so important to him. The routine, the familiarity and the prospect of even a fleeting sense of improvement helped him to maintain a connection with himself as his health rapidly declined. He never failed to send me a message after each treatment. I still have the last one he ever sent:

Thank you, dear Gerad. I feel marvellous as I always do after a session but today was special. It was like a drug hit! I look forward to more. Yours, John.

EPILOGUE

*

The stories in this book are not just about transformation. They are about seeing ourselves through an entirely different lens, one that challenges conventional narratives about health and wellbeing. By sharing the journeys of my patients, my aim has been to show you what is possible when we free ourselves from the beliefs that bind us and align ourselves with Nature instead.

In the West, we are told to search for the roots of our suffering in our upbringing, our environment, our relationships, or our biology. Five-Element Acupuncture goes deeper, moving beyond the circumstances of our lives to examine the very substance from which we are made. The five elements are not abstract or mystical. On the contrary, they are the origin of all life, so when one of them loses its natural state of balance, it is hardly surprising that there are consequences.

Take Tarik, for example. He came to me with a variety of symptoms but had no awareness of the anger and frustration that permeated his every thought and action. He had spent years trying to understand why he struggled,

EPILOGUE

yet it never occurred to him to look within. Instead, he blamed his suffering on his childhood and the neglect of those who were meant to nurture him. Through the lens of the five elements, however, it was clear that his Wood element was struggling to fulfil its natural remit of renewal and growth. The inevitable outcome was an inability to realise his own potential, leaving him paralysed by fury and alienated from everyone around him.

In the same way, Martha was a prisoner of her past. She arrived in my clinic feeling hollow and disconnected, as though she were a ghost in her own life. She was deeply resentful, having convinced herself that her unhappiness was the result of failed relationships and unmet expectations. In truth, it was the consequence of an imbalance in the Metal element that deprived her of freshness of spirit and the capacity to forgive and let go.

These stories remind us that healing is not about fixing what is broken; it is about restoring our natural equilibrium, which in turn ignites the possibility of profound transformation and the discovery of our true essence. My hope is that they will inspire you to look at yourself and those around you through new eyes, for beneath our struggles and our stories lies a deeper truth: we are all an exquisite interplay of the five elements, striving for balance, yearning for harmony. When we embrace this understanding, we open ourselves to healing – not only of our symptoms, but of our lives.

GLOSSARY

Qi
A concept from traditional Chinese culture that refers to the vital life force or energy that flows through the entire universe and all living things.

The Five Elements
Five-Element Acupuncture understands the universe as being composed of five expressions of Qi: Water, Wood, Fire, Earth, and Metal. Health arises when these elements are in balance. When they are not, physical, mental, or emotional symptoms appear. Treatment restores harmony by diagnosing the root imbalance and using fine needles and/or warmth (moxa) at acupuncture points to affect the flow and restore the strength of qi.

Officials
An ancient analogy used in Chinese medicine describes the organs and functions of the body as "Officials," each with their own specific responsibility, much like ministers in a royal court. Together, they maintain the overall balance and health of the person.

Causative Factor (CF)
The Causative Factor is the core elemental imbalance in a person – the root cause of all disharmony in their body, mind, and spirit. By treating the CF, the body's innate ability to rebalance, heal and transform is restored.

Meridians
Meridians are the energetic pathways through which Qi flows throughout the body, mind, and spirit. Each is associated with a specific organ-function (Official) and is interconnected with the others.

Acupuncture Points
These are precise locations on the meridians where Qi can be accessed and influenced. Each point has unique properties and is chosen for its effect on balancing the elements and restoring harmony.

Chinese Pulses
The Chinese pulses are found just above the radial artery at the wrist – six on each side – corresponding to the twelve Officials. In a state of balance, each pulse re!ects the Officials sharing the body's energy equally and harmoniously.

A GUIDE TO THE FIVE ELEMENTS

Wood
- **Season:** Spring
- **Emotion:** Anger (and assertiveness or frustration)
- **Organs** (Officials):
  – Liver: responsible for planning
  – Gall Bladder: responsible for decisions/actions

Fire
- **Season:** Summer
- **Emotion:** Joy (or lack thereof)
- **Organs** (Officials):
  – Heart: responsible for the overall control of all the Officials
  – Small Intestine: responsible for sorting the pure from the impure
  – Circulation/Sex: responsible for the free circulation of Qi, sexual secretions and protection of the heart
  – Three Heater – responsible for regulation and temperature control

Earth
- **Season:** Late summer*
- **Emotion:** Sympathy (and worry/ a need to be understood)
- **Organs** (Officials):
  – Spleen: responsible for all transportation
  – Stomach: responsible for processing (rotting and ripening)

Metal
- **Season:** Autumn
- **Emotion:** Grief (letting go or holding on)
- **Organs** (Officials):
  – Lung: responsible for receiving the heavenly Qi
  – Large intestine: responsible for the elimination of waste

Water
- **Season:** Winter
- **Emotion:** Fear (or lack thereof)
- **Organs** (Officials):
  – Kidney: responsible for the control of the waterways
  – Bladder: responsible for the maintenance of the reservoirs

In ancient Chinese cosmology, the seasonal cycle includes a fifth season – Late Summer – associated with Earth, a time of harvest and transformation.

GERAD KITE is a master of Five-Element Acupuncture and the founder of Kite Clinic in London where he has empowered thousands of people to tap into the truth of who they really are. He is also the founder of Yellow Path acupuncture school and the bestselling author of *Everything You Need You Have* and *The Art of Baby Making*.

JAMES EDEN has worked in storytelling for more than thirty years, firstly as a producer in the world of advertising and film production, and latterly as a writer. He has a degree in modern languages and is a lifelong student of Eastern philosophy.